D1136442

# Springer

*Berlin*
*Heidelberg*
*New York*
*Barcelona*
*Budapest*
*Hong Kong*
*London*
*Milan*
*Paris*
*Santa Clara*
*Singapore*
*Tokyo*

# UICC
International Union Against Cancer
Union Internationale Contre le Cancer

P. Hermanek · R. V. P. Hutter · L. H. Sobin ·
G. Wagner · Ch. Wittekind (Eds.)

# TNM Atlas

Illustrated Guide
to the TNM/pTNM Classification
of Malignant Tumours

Edited by
P. Hermanek    R.V. P. Hutter    L.H. Sobin    G. Wagner    Ch. Wittekind

Fourth Edition

With 479 illustrations and an insert with summaries
of the T and N defintions by site

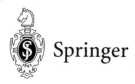

Springer

P. Hermanek
Universität Erlangen-Nürnberg
Chirurgische Universitätsklinik Erlangen
Krankenhausstraße 12, D-91054 Erlangen

R. V. P. Hutter
University of Medicine and
Dentistry New Jersey
New Jersey Medical School
Dept. of Pathology
Saint Barnabas Medical Center
Old Short Hills Road,
Livingston, NJ 07039, USA

L. H. Sobin
Division of Gastrointenstinal Pathology
Armed Forces Institute of Pathology
Washington DC 20306, USA

G. Wagner
Deutsches Krebsforschungszentrum
Heidelberg
Institut für Epidemiologie und Biometrie
Im Neuenheimer Feld 280,
D-69120 Heidelberg

Ch. Wittekind
Institut für Pathologie
Universität Leipzig
Liebigstraße 26, D-04103 Leipzig

1st Edition 1982; 2nd Edition 1985; 3rd Edition 1989
3rd Edition, Corrected Reprint 1990; 3rd Edition, 2nd Revision 1992

ISBN 3-540-62704-9
4th edition Springer-Verlag Berlin Heidelberg New York

Die Deutsche Bibliothek – CIP-Einheitsaufnahme

TNM atlas: illustrated guide to the TNM/pTNM classification of malignant tumours/UICC,
International Union against Cancer. P. Hermanek ... – 4. ed. – Berlin; Heidelberg; New York;
Barcelona; Budapest; Hong Kong; London; Milan; Paris; Santa Clara; Singapore; Tokyo:
Springer, 1997
     ISBN 3-540-62704-9

Cover design: Erich Kirchner
Illustrations: P. Lübke
Typesetting: Michael Kusche, Goldener Schnitt

SPIN-Nr. 10670132     19/3111     – 5 4 3 2 – Printed on acid-free paper

# Preface to the Fourth Edition

This new fourth edition of the *TNM Atlas* reflects the changes in the TNM system introduced by the recently published fifth edition of the *TNM Classification of Malignant Tumours* [1]. The most important additions and modifications are:

- A revised classification of nasopharyngeal carcinoma reflecting the needs of radiation oncologists
- Changes in the regional lymph node classification of gastric carcinoma
- Expansion of the soft tissue tumour classification
- A new classification of fallopian tube carcinoma and of gestational trophoblastic tumours
- A revised testis tumour classification
- Important changes in the classification of prostate and urinary bladder tumours reflecting advances in urology

The editorial board has changed: Dr. Spiessl, the editor-in-chief and "father" of the *TNM Atlas*, has retired, as have Dr. Beahrs and Dr. Scheibe; Dr. Wittekind has joined. The editors wish to express many thanks to Bernd Spiessl for his great contributions to the development and promotion of the *TNM Atlas*. We are grateful to Dr. Beahrs and Dr. Scheibe for their work on the editorial board as well as for their other TNM activities.

The editorial board has tried to follow the successful concept developed by Bernd Spiessl to provide a graphic aid for the practical application of the TNM classification system. The TNM classification, as presented and illustrated in this edition, corresponds exactly to the fifth edition of the UICC *TNM Classification of Malignant Tumours* [1] and the fifth edition of the AJCC *Cancer Staging Manual* [2]. Recent modifications by FIGO [3] are also included in order to keep the FIGO and TNM classifications identical.

Substantial changes between the revised third edition (1992) and the present edition of the *TNM Atlas* are indicated by a line at the left-hand side of the page.

The editors hope that the *TNM Atlas* will continue to facilitate the daily practice of oncologists and to enhance the use of TNM in planning treatment, estimating prognosis and evaluating treatment results.

July 1997

P. Hermanek, Erlangen
R. V. P. Hutter, Livingston, NJ
L. H. Sobin, Washington, DC
G. Wagner, Heidelberg
Ch. Wittekind, Leipzig

# References

1. Sobin LH, Wittekind Ch (eds) (1997) UICC: TNM Classification of Malignant Tumours, 5th edition. John Wiley, New York
2. Fleming ID, Cooper JS, Henson DE, Hutter RVP, Kennedy BJ, Murphy GP, O´Sullivan B, Sobin LH, Yarbro JW (eds) (1997) AJCC: Cancer Staging Manual, 5th edition. Lippincott-Raven, Philadelphia
3. Pettersson F (ed) (1995) FIGO: Annual report on the results of treatment in gynecological cancer, vol 22. Radiumhemmet, Stockholm

# Preface to the Third Edition

In 1938 the League of Nations Health Organization published an *Atlas Illustrating the Division of Cancer of the Uterine Cervix into Four Stages* (edited by J. Heymann, Stockholm). Since this work appeared, the idea of visual representation of the anatomical extent of malignant tumours at the different stages of their development has been repeatedly discussed.

At its meeting in Copenhagen in July 1954, the UICC adopted as part of its programme "the realization of a clinical atlas". However, the time to publish the planned book of illustrations was not ripe until the national committees and international organizations had officially recognized the 28 classifications of malignant tumours at various sites as presented in the third edition of the *TNM Booklet* edited by M. Harmer *(TNM Classification of Malignant Tumours, 1978).* This was all the more important since publication of the Booklet was followed in 1980 by publication of *A Brochure of Checklists,* edited by A. H. Sellers, a further aid in the practical application of the TNM system.

The *TNM Atlas* (first edition 1982, second edition 1985) was the third of the aids intended to fulfil the one ultimate purpose of making the classification of the anatomical extent of malignant tumours as much a routine procedure as histological typing and grading.

A strong interest in the *TNM Atlas* manifested itself in the unexpectedly large demand for copies. Its strength in publicizing the use of the TNM system is encouraging and demonstrates the urgency of making the abbreviations of tumour findings easily understandable. The busy doctor is then in a position to comprehend at a glance not only the principle of the system, but also to put together easily the correct finding formulations in individual cases.

The public aimed at by the *Atlas* is, in the first instance, those doctors working in the field of oncology who should be interested in the general acceptance and use of the TNM rules. These rules are considered to be an internationally accepted, uniform, generally binding and understood system which describes tumour stages exactly and thus facilitates the collection and the exchange of comparable data.

The third edition of the *TNM Classification of Malignant Tumours* appeared in 1978. Since then, the diagnosis of tumours has made great progress thanks to the wide application of computer tomography and through the introduction of endoscopic sonography and nuclear magnetic resonance imaging. Different studies have resulted in new knowledge about the relationship between the extent of the tumour at the time of diagnosis and the later course of disease.

As can be ascertained, some users of the TNM system changed the official definitions according to their own conceptions. In order to counteract this development and in order to take into account the scientific progress of the last 10 years, the national TNM committees agreed in 1982 to revise the 1978 *TNM Classification* and also to introduce new classifications for organs which had not yet been considered in the TNM system. The desired objective is to once again create generally accepted and internationally unified rules.

This objective was attained in 1986 after numerous national and international meetings. The result of these meetings – the fourth edition of the international *TNM Classification,* which was accepted by the TNM Committee of the UICC – was published in English in the spring of 1987.[1]

Malignant tumours of the following organs were newly classified:
- Head and neck: Salivary glands and maxillary sinus
- Gastrointestinal tract: Liver, gallbladder, extrahepatic biliary ducts, ampulla of Vater, pancreas
- Urological tumours: Renal pelvis and ureter, urethra
- Bones
- Brain

In the fourth edition, the TNM classification of gynaecological tumours coincides with the classification of the Federation Internationale de Gynécologie et d´Obstétrique (FIGO). The classification of paediatric tumours is identical to that of the Sociéte Internationale d'Oncologie Pédiatrique (SIOP). The definitions which appear in the fourth edition were accepted by all national TNM committees including the American Joint Committee on Cancer (AJCC), so that now an internationally unified, up-to-date classification of tumours by anatomical extent is at our disposal.

The publication of the fourth edition of the *TNM Classification* necessitated the revision of the *TNM Atlas.* The present, third edition of the *TNM Atlas* takes into consideration all the additions and changes made in the fourth edition of the *TNM Classification* and, therefore, represents the current state of TNM classification as accepted world-wide by all the national committees and as it appears in the third edition of the *AJCC Manual for Staging of Cancer* (1988).

---

[1]    UICC: TNM Classification of Malignant Tumours, 4th edn. P. Hermanek, L. H. Sobin (eds) (1987) Springer, Berlin Heidelberg New York London Paris Tokyo

The editorial board was expanded by the inclusion of the Chairman of the TNM Project Committee of the UICC, L. H. Sobin, as well as two representatives of the AJCC.

The third edition of the *TNM Atlas* follows the sound principles on which previous editions were based. The structure of the *TNM Atlas* is similar to that of the *TNM Classification*. The Atlas´ text is limited to the essentials, so that the original *Booklet* should be consulted for detailed information, principles and general rules of the TNM system.

For practical reasons, the format chosen is as similar as possible to that of the *TNM Booklet*. The one is not supposed to replace but rather to supplement the other. A major aim of the *TNM Atlas* is, therefore, to promote understanding of and interest in the application of the TNM system and to show how simply, uniformly and precisely the system is structured.

January 1989

B. Spiessl, Basel
O. H. Beahrs, Rochester, Minn
P. Hermanek, Erlangen
R. V. P. Hutter, Livingston, NJ
O. Scheibe, Stuttgart
L. H. Sobin, Washington, DC
G. Wagner, Heidelberg

# Foreword to the First Edition

Confronted with a myriad of T´s, N´s and M´s in the UICC TNM booklet, classifying a malignancy may seem to many cancer clinicians a tedious, dull and pedantic task. But with a look at the *TNM Atlas* all of a sudden lifeless categories become vivid images, challenging the clinicians´s know-how and investigational skills.

Rotterdam, July 1982

Birgit van der Werf-Messing, M. D.
Professor of Radiology
Chairman of the International
TNM-Committee of the UICC

# Acknowledgements

The editors wish to express their thanks to Mrs. J. Wagner, Erlangen, for her help with the preparation of the manuscript. They are equally grateful to Mrs. U. Kerl-Jentzsch, Mr. J. Kühn, Mr. M. Hasse and Mr. P. Lübke, who took great care in drawing the anatomical illustrations.

Financial support for the publication of the first and second edition of the TNM Atlas was provided by the Federal Ministry of Science and Technology, Bonn. The editors are indebted to this authority. Support of the TNM Project by the Centers for Disease Control and Prevention (USA) through grants R13/CC R012626-01 is gratefully acknowledged.

Finally, the editors wish to thank Springer-Verlag and its staff for their speedy handling of the matter as well as for the excellent presentation of this *Atlas*.

# Contributors of the Fourth Edition

Bootz F., Leipzig, FRG — Head and neck surgery

Hermanek P., Erlangen, FRG — Pathology

Howaldt H. J., Gießen, FRG — Head and neck surgery

Hutter R. V. P., Livingston, NJ, USA — Pathology

Paterok E., Erlangen, FRG — Gynaecology

Sobin L. H., Washington, DC, USA — Pathology

Wagner G., Heidelberg, FRG — Documentation and Epidemiology

Wittekind Ch., Leipzig, FRG — Pathology

# Contributors to the Third Edition

| | |
|---|---|
| Baker, H. W., Portland, Ore, USA | Head and neck surgery |
| Beahrs, O. H., Rochester, Minn, USA | General surgery |
| Drepper, H., Münster-Handorf, FRG | Maxillofacial surgery |
| Gemsenjäger, E., Basel, Switzerland | General surgery |
| Genz, T., Berlin | Gynaecology |
| Glanz, H., Marburg, FRG | Otorhinolaryngology |
| Hasse, J., Freiburg, FRG | Thoracic surgery |
| Hermanek, P., Erlangen, FRG | Pathology |
| Hutter, R. V. P., Livingston, NJ, USA | Pathology |
| Kindermann, G., München, FRG | Gynaecology |
| Kleinsasser, O., Marburg, FRG | Otorhinolaryngology |
| Lang, G., Erlangen, FRG | Ophthalmology |
| Naumann, G. O. H., Erlangen, FRG | Ophthalmology |
| Remagen, W., Basel, Switzerland | Pathology |
| Scheibe, O., Stuttgart, FRG | General surgery |
| Schmitt, H. P., Heidelberg, FRG | Neuropathology |
| Sobin, L. H., Washington, DC, USA | Pathology |
| Spiessl, B., Basel, Switzerland | Maxillofacial surgery |
| Wagner, G., Heidelberg, FRG | Documentation and Epidemiology |

# Contributors to the Second Edition

| | |
|---|---|
| Adolphs, H. D., Höxter, FRG | Urology |
| Amberger, H., Heidelberg, FRG | General surgery |
| Baumann, R. P., Neuchâtel, Switzerland | Pathology |
| Berger, H., Göttingen, FRG | Dermatology |
| Bokelmann, D., Essen, FRG | General surgery |
| Brandeis, W. F., Heidelberg, FRG | Paediatric oncology |
| Dold, U., Gauting, FRG | Internal medicine |
| Drepper, H., Münster-Handorf, FRG | Maxillofacial surgery |
| Drings, P., Heidelberg, FRG | Internal medicine |
| Gemsenjäger, E., Basel, Switzerland | General surgery |
| Hasse, J., Basel, Switzerland | Thoracic surgery |
| Heitz, Ph., Basel, Switzerland | Pathology |
| Hermanek, P., Erlangen, FRG | Pathology |
| Karrer, K., Wien, Austria | Oncological epidemiology |
| Kuehnl-Petzold, C. Freiburg i.Br., FRG | Dermatology |
| Liebenstein, J., Mannheim, FRG | Gynaecology |
| Molitor, D., Bonn, FRG | Urology |
| Nidecker, A., Basel, Switzerland | Radiology |
| Rohde, H., Köln FRG | General surgery |
| Scheibe, O., Stuttgart, FRG | General surgery |
| Schmitt, A., Mannheim, FRG | Gynaecology |
| Spiessl, B., Basel, Switzerland | Maxillofacial surgery |
| Thomas, C., Marburg, FRG | Pathology |
| Vogt-Moykopf, I., Heidelberg, FRG | Thoracic surgery |
| Wagner, G., Heidelberg, FRG | Documentation and Epidemiology |

# Contents

# Preliminary Note[1]

The TNM system for describing the anatomical extent of disease is based on the assessment of three components:

T – The extent of the *primary tumour*
N – The absence or presence and extent of *regional lymph node metastasis*
M – The absence or presence of *distant metastasis*

The addition of numbers to these three components indicates the extent of the malignant disease, thus:

T0, T1, T2, T3, T4   N0, N1, N2, N3   M0, M1

In effect, the system is a „shorthand notation" for describing the extent of a particular malignant tumour.

Each site is described under the following headings:

1. *Anatomy*. Drawings of the anatomical sites and subsites are presented with the appropriate ICD-O topography numbers.[1]
2. *Regional Lymph Nodes*. The regional lymph nodes are listed and shown in drawings.
3. *T/pT Clinical and Pathological Classification of the Primary Tumour*. Above all, the definitions for T and pT categories are presented. Because in the fifth edition of the TNM Classification the clinical and pathological classification (T and pT) generally coincide, the same illustrations are valid for the T and pT classification. The only exception to this is the retinoblastoma.
4. *N/pN Clinical and Pathological Classification of Regional Lymph Nodes*. The N and pN categories are presented in a fashion similar to the T and pT categories. Differences between N and pN definitions in the fifth edition arise only in the case of carcinoma of the breast and germinal tumours of the testis.
5. *M/pM Clinical and Pathological Classification of Distant Metastasis*. The presentation of the many possible variables of the M localization is given only in some selected cases.

---

[1] ICD-O International Classification of Diseases for Oncology, 2nd edn (1990) WHO, Geneva

## C-Factor

The C-factor, or certainty factor, reflects the validity of classification according to the diagnostic methods employed. Its use is optional. The C-factor definitions are:

C1    Evidence from standard diagnostic means (e.g. inspection, palpation and standard radiography, intraluminal endoscopy for tumours of certain organs)

C2    Evidence obtained by special diagnostic means [e.g. radiographic imaging in special projections, tomography, computerized tomography (CT), ultrasonography, lymphography, angiography; scintigraphy; magnetic resonance imaging (MRI); endoscopy, biopsy, and cytology]

C3    Evidence from surgical exploration, including biopsy and cytology

C4    Evidence of the extent of disease following definitive surgery and pathological examination of the resected specimen

C5    Evidence from autopsy

**Example:** Degrees of C may be applied to the T, N and M categories. A case might be described as T3C2, N2C1, M0C2.

The TNM clinical classification is, therefore, equivalent to C1, C2 and C3 in varying degrees of certainty, while the pTNM pathological classification generally is equivalent to C4.

## Residual Tumour (R) Classification

The absence or presence of residual tumour after treatment is described by the symbol R. Its use is optional.

TNM and pTNM describe the anatomical extent of cancer in general without considering treatment. They can be supplemented by the R classification, which deals with tumour status after treatment. The R classification reflects the effects of therapy, influences further therapeutic procedures and is a strong predictor of prognosis.

In the R classification, not only local-regional residual tumour is to be taken into consideration, but also distant residual tumour in the form of remaining distant metastases.

The definitions of the R categories are:

RX    Presence of residual tumour cannot be assessed

R0    No residual tumour (Fig. 1)

R1    Microscopic residual tumour (Fig. 2)

R2    Macroscopic residual tumour (Fig. 3)

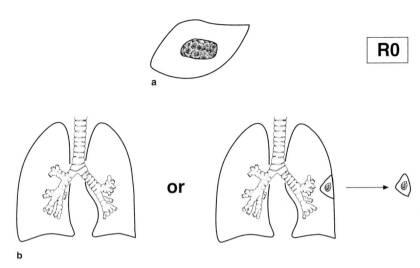

**Fig. 1a–c.** R0. **a** Primary tumour excised, resection margins without tumour. **b** No distant metastasis or distant metastasis completely removed

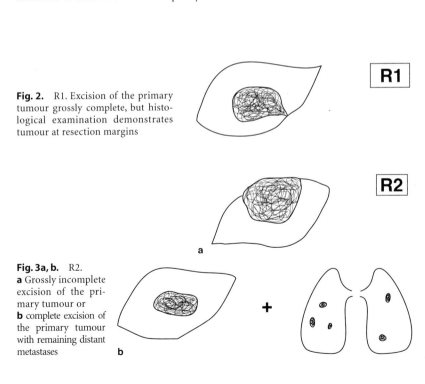

**Fig. 2.** R1. Excision of the primary tumour grossly complete, but histological examination demonstrates tumour at resection margins

**Fig. 3a, b.** R2. **a** Grossly incomplete excision of the primary tumour or **b** complete excision of the primary tumour with remaining distant metastases

# Head and Neck Tumours

## Introductory Notes

The following sites are included:

Lip, oral cavity
Pharynx: Oropharynx, nasopharynx, hypopharynx
Larynx: Supraglottis, glottis, subglottis
Maxillary and ethmoid sinus
Salivary glands
Thyroid gland

Substantial changes in the fourth edition of 1997 compared to the revised third edition of 1992 are marked by a line at the left-hand side of the page. The same is true for new classifications of previously unclassified tumours.

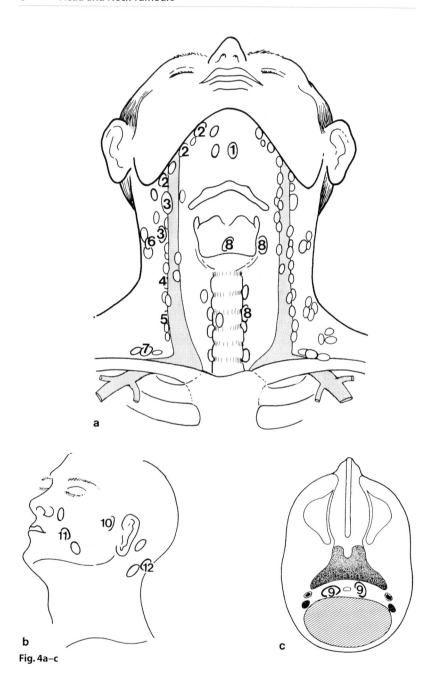

a

b

c

**Fig. 4a–c**

## Regional Lymph Nodes (Fig. 4)

The regional lymph nodes for all head and neck sites except nasopharynx and thyroid are the cervical nodes. These include

 (1) submental nodes
 (2) submandibular nodes
 (3) cranial jugular (deep cervical) nodes
 (4) medial jugular (deep cervical) nodes
 (5) caudal jugular (deep cervical) nodes
 (6) dorsal cervical (superficial cervical) nodes along the accessory nerve
 (7) supraclavicular nodes
 (8) prelaryngeal and paratracheal nodes
 (9) retropharyngeal nodes
(10) parotid nodes
(11) buccal nodes
(12) retroauricular and occipital nodes

## N/pN Classification

The definitions of the N and pN categories for all head and neck sites except nasopharynx and thyroid gland are:

## N/pN – Regional Lymph Nodes

N/pNX    Regional lymph nodes cannot be assessed
N/pN0    No regional lymph node metastasis

pN0      Histological examination of a selective neck dissection specimen will ordinarily include 6 or more lymph nodes. Histological examination of a radical or modified radical neck dissection specimen will ordinarily include 10 or more lymph nodes.

N/pN1    Metastasis in a single ipsilateral lymph node, 3 cm or less in greatest
dimension (Fig. 5)

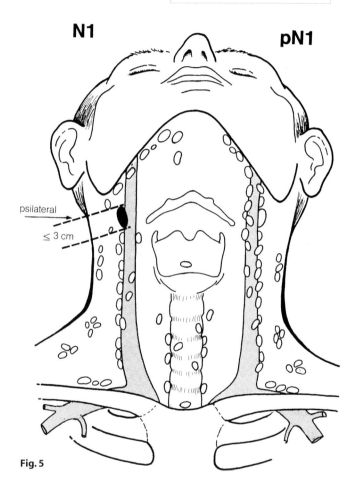

**Fig. 5**

N/pN2  Metastasis in a single ipsilateral lymph node, more than 3 cm but not more than 6 cm in greatest dimension; or in multiple ipsilateral lymph nodes, none more than 6 cm in greatest dimension; or in bilateral or contralateral lymph nodes, none more than 6 cm in greatest dimension

N/pN2a  Metastasis in a single ipsilateral lymph node, more than 3 cm but not more than 6 cm in greatest dimension (Fig. 6)

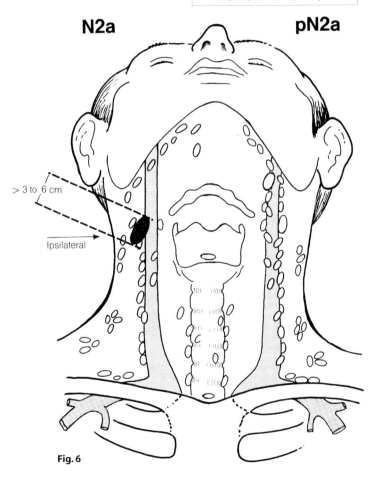

Any head or neck primary except nasopharynx and thyroid gland

**N2a**

**pN2a**

> 3 to 6 cm

Ipsilateral

**Fig. 6**

N/pN2b  Metastasis in multiple ipsilateral lymph nodes, none more than 6 cm in greatest dimension (Fig. 7)

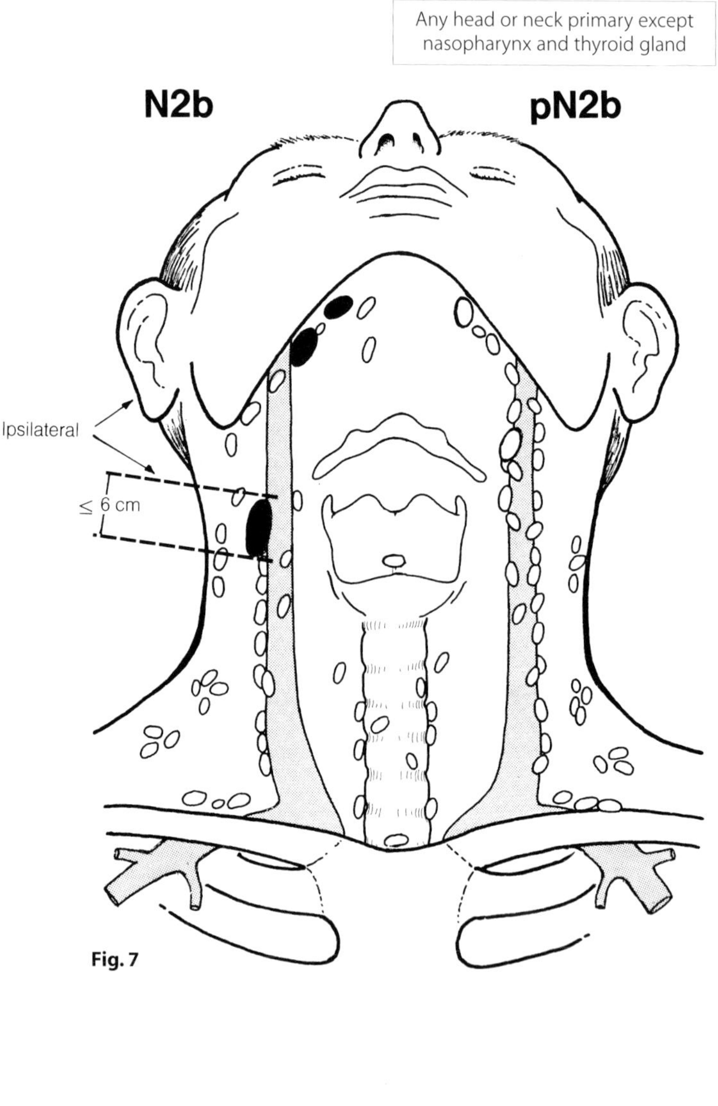

**N2b**    **pN2b**

Any head or neck primary except nasopharynx and thyroid gland

Ipsilateral

≤ 6 cm

**Fig. 7**

N/pN2c  Metastasis in bilateral or contralateral lymph nodes, none more than 6 cm in greatest dimension (Fig. 8)

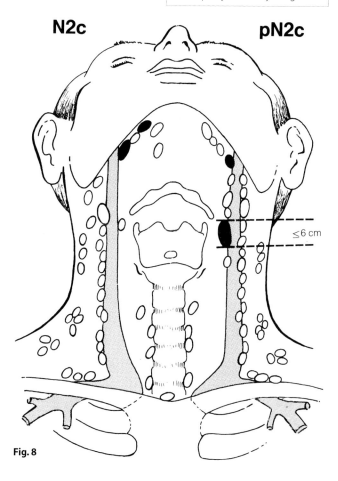

Any head or neck primary except nasopharynx and thyroid gland

**N2c**                    **pN2c**

≤6 cm

**Fig. 8**

N/pN3    Metastasis in a lymph node, more than 6 cm in greatest dimension (Fig. 9)

**Note:**    Midline nodes are considered ipsilateral nodes.

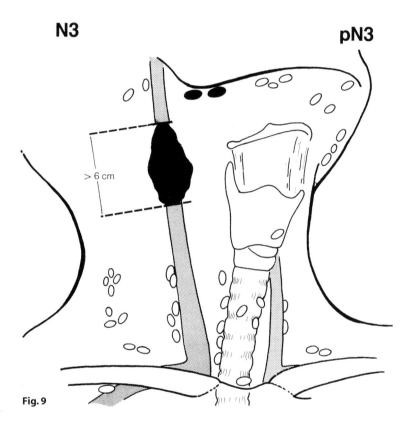

Fig. 9

# Lip and Oral Cavity (ICD-O C00, C02-C06)

## Rules for Classification

The classification applies only to carcinomas of the vermilion surfaces of the lips and of the oral cavity, including those of minor salivary glands. There should be histological confirmation of the disease.

## Anatomical Sites and Subsites

*Lip* (Fig. 10)

1. External upper lip (vermilion border) (C00.0)
2. External lower lip (vermilion border) (C00.1)
3. Commissures (C00.6)

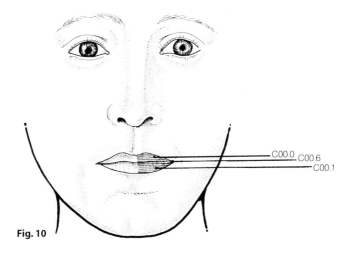

**Fig. 10**

*Oral Cavity* (Figs. 11–13)

1. Buccal mucosa
   i)    Mucosa of upper and lower lips (C00.3, 4)
   ii)   Cheek mucosa (C06.0)
   iii) Retromolar areas (C06.2)
   iv) Bucco-alveolar sulci, upper and lower (vestibule of mouth) (C06.1)
2. Upper alveolus and gingiva (upper gum) (C03.0)
3. Lower alveolus and gingiva (lower gum) (C03.1)
4. Hard palate (C05.0)
5. Tongue
   i)    Dorsal surface and lateral borders anterior to vallate papillae (anterior two-thirds) (C02.0,1)
   ii)   Inferior (ventral) surface (C02.2)
6. Floor of mouth (C04)

**Note:** Base of tongue (C01.9) belongs to pharynx (see pp. 22, 23).

# Regional Lymph Nodes

See p. 7.

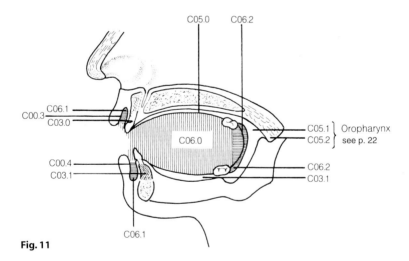

**Fig. 11**

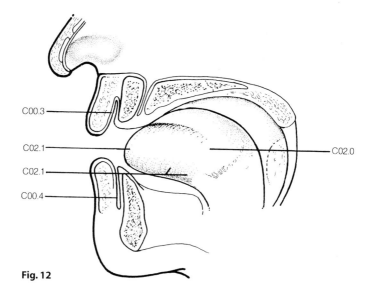

C00.3
C02.1
C02.1
C00.4
C02.0

**Fig. 12**

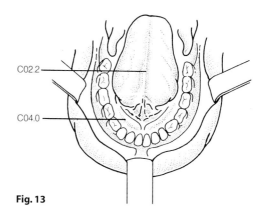

C02.2
C04.0

**Fig. 13**

## TN Clinical Classification

### T – Primary Tumour

TX     Primary tumour cannot be assessed
T0     No evidence of primary tumour
Tis    Carcinoma in situ


T1     Tumour 2 cm or less in greatest dimension (Figs. 14, 15)
T2     Tumour more than 2 cm but not more than 4 cm in greatest dimension (Figs. 16, 17)
T3     Tumour more than 4 cm in greatest dimension (Figs. 18, 19)

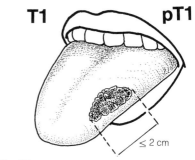

**Fig. 14**

**Fig. 15**

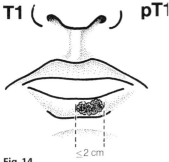
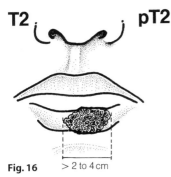
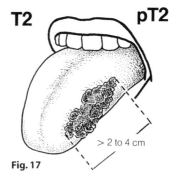

**Fig. 16**     > 2 to 4 cm

**Fig. 17**

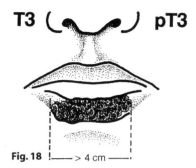

T3 ( ) pT3

Fig. 18    ——— > 4 cm ———

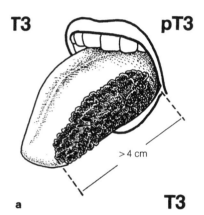

T3        pT3

> 4 cm

a

T3

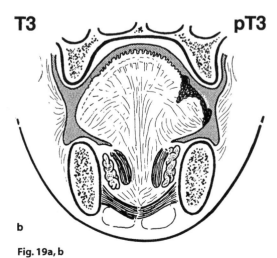

T3        pT3

b

Fig. 19a, b

T4     **Lip:** Tumour invades adjacent structures, e.g. through cortical bone, infe-
       rior alveolar nerve, floor of mouth, skin of face (Figs. 20, 21)
       **Oral Cavity:** Tumour invades adjacent structures, e.g. through cortical
       bone, into deep (extrinsic) muscle of tongue, maxillary sinus, skin (Figs.
       22–24)

**Notes:**   1. The extrinsic musculature of the tongue includes musculi hyo-, stylo-, genio-
       and palatoglossus. Invasion of the intrinsic muscle alone (musculi longitudi-
       nales superior and inferior, transversus linguae and verticalis linguae) is not
       classified T4 (Fig. 19b).
       2. Superficial erosion alone of bone/tooth socket by gingival primary is not suf-
       ficient to classify a tumour as T4.
       3. In cases of doubt regarding the invasion through cortical bone, such as that
       of Fig. 23a, paragraph 4 of the General Rules of the TNM System (TNM
       Booklet, p. 7) should be applied: „If there is doubt concerning the correct T, N
       or M category to which a particular case should be allotted, the lower (i.e. less
       advanced) category should be chosen. This will also be reflected in the stage
       grouping". If scintigraphy is feasible and the resultant finding is conclusive as
       shown in Fig. 23b, the tumour must be classified as T4.

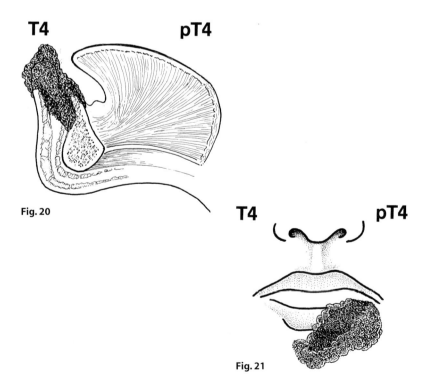

**T4**          **pT4**

**Fig. 20**

**T4**          **pT4**

**Fig. 21**

**T4**                                                    **pT4**

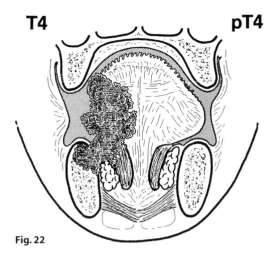

**Fig. 22**

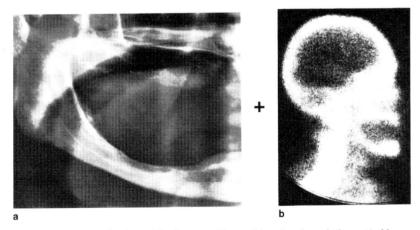

a                                                         b

**Fig. 23.** **a** Radiographical suspicion but no evidence of invasion through the cortical bone; the tumour must be classified as non-T4 in correspondence with the definitions T1, T2 and T3. **b** Evidence of invasion through cortical bone by uptake, which corresponds with the suspected area in the premolar region of the radiograph shown in a. On the basis of the scintigraphic finding the tumour must be classified as T4

**T4**

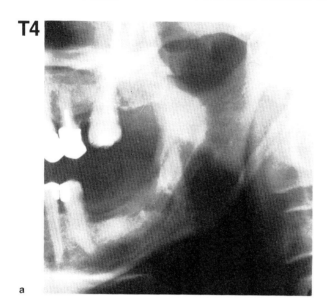

a

**T4**

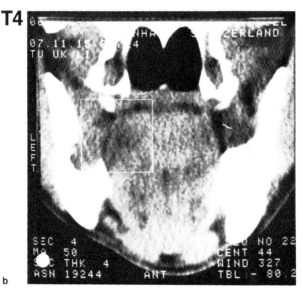

b

**Fig. 24.**  **a** Evidence of invasion through cortical bone of the mandibula. **b** CT of case shown in a. The carcinoma of the floor of the mouth invades through the cortical bone and into the extrinsic muscle of the tongue (m. hyoglossus)

## N – Regional Lymph Nodes

See p. 7.

## pTN Pathological Classification

The pT and pN categories correspond to the T and N categories.

# Pharynx (ICD-O C01.9, C05.1,2, CO9, C10.0,2,3, C11-13)

## Rules for Classification

The classification applies only to carcinomas. There should be histological confirmation of the disease.

## Anatomical Sites and Subsites

**Oropharynx** (C01.9, C05.1,2, C09.0,1,9, C10.0,2,3) (Figs. 25, 26)

1. Anterior wall (glosso-epiglottic area)
   i)   Base of tongue (posterior to the vallate papillae or posterior third) (C01.9)
   ii)  Vallecula (C10.0)
2. Lateral wall (C10.2)
   i)   Tonsil (C09.9)
   ii)  Tonsillar fossa (C09.0) and tonsillar (faucial) pillars (C09.1)
   iii) Glossotonsillar sulci (tonsillar pillars) (C09.1)
3. Posterior wall (C10.3)
4. Superior wall
   i)   Inferior surface of soft palate (C05.1)
   ii)  Uvula(C05.2)

**Note:** The lingual (anterior) surface of the epiglottis (C10.1) is included with the larynx, suprahyoid epiglottis.

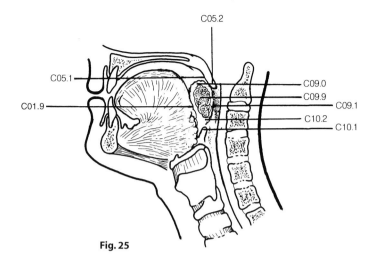

**Fig. 25**

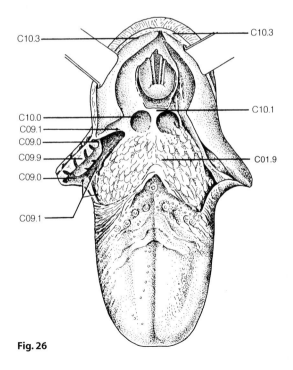

**Fig. 26**

## Nasopharynx (C11) (Fig. 27)

1. Postero-superior wall: extends from the level of the junction of the hard and soft palates to the base of the skull (C11.0,1)
2. Lateral wall: includes the fossa of Rosenmüller (C11.2)
3. Inferior wall: consists of the superior surface of the soft palate (C11.3)

**Note:** The margin of the choanal orifices, including the posterior margin of the nasal septum, is included with the nasal fossa.

## Hypopharynx (C12, C13) (Fig. 27)

1. Pharyngo-oesophageal junction (postcricoid area) (C13.0): extends from the level of the arytenoid cartilages and connecting folds to the inferior border of the cricoid cartilage, thus forming the anterior wall of the hypopharynx
2. Piriform sinus (C12.9): extends from the pharyngo-epiglottic fold to the upper end of the oesophagus. It is bounded laterally by the thyroid cartilage and medially by the hypopharyngeal surface of the aryepiglottic fold (C13.1) and the arytenoid and cricoid cartilages
3. Posterior pharyngeal wall (C13.2): extends from the superior level of the hyoid bone (or floor of the vallecula) to the level of the inferior border of the cricoid cartilage and from the apex of one piriform sinus to the other

## Regional Lymph Nodes

See p. 7.

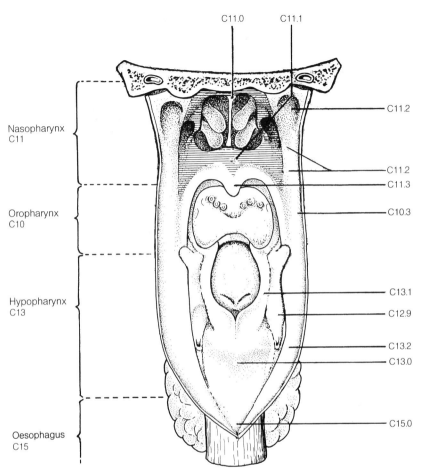

**Fig. 27**

## TN Clinical Classification

### T – Primary Tumour

TX    Primary tumour cannot be assessed
T0    No evidence of primary tumour
Tis    Carcinoma in situ

#### *Oropharynx*

T1    Tumour 2 cm or less in greatest dimension (Fig. 28)
T2    Tumour more than 2 cm but not more than 4 cm in greatest dimension (Fig. 29)
T3    Tumour more than 4 cm in greatest dimension (Fig. 30)
T4    Tumour invades adjacent structures, e.g. pterygoid muscles, mandible, hard palate, deep muscle of tongue (Fig. 31), larynx

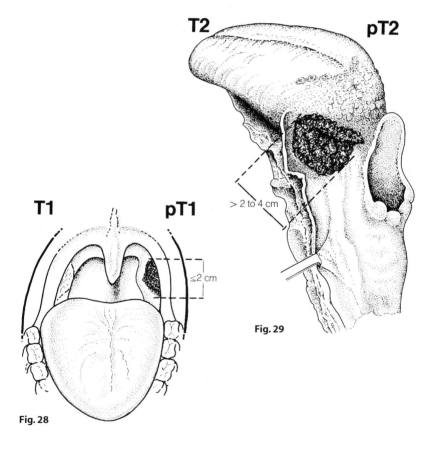

**Fig. 29**

**Fig. 28**

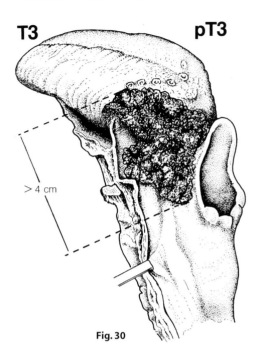

T3    pT3

> 4 cm

**Fig. 30**

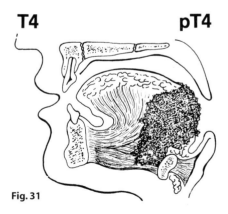

T4    pT4

**Fig. 31**

## Nasopharynx

T1    Tumour confined to nasopharynx (Fig. 32)
T2    Tumour extends to soft tissue of oropharynx and/or nasal fossa (Fig. 32)
    T2a    without parapharyngeal extension[1] (Fig. 33)
    T2b    with parapharyngeal extension[1] (Fig. 34)
T3    Tumour invades bony structures and/or paranasal sinuses (Fig. 35)
T4    Tumour with intracranial extension and/or involvement of cranial ner-
    ves, infratemporal fossa, hypopharynx, or orbit (Figs. 36, 37)

**Note:**    1. Parapharyngeal extension denotes postero-lateral infiltration of tumour
    beyond the pharyngo-basilar fascia.

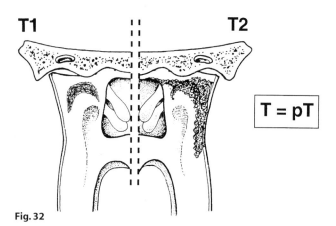

**T1**                                    **T2**

T = pT

**Fig. 32**

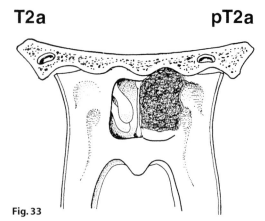

**T2a**                          **pT2a**

**Fig. 33**

**T2b**                                        **pT2b**

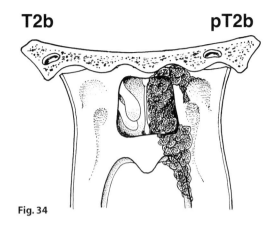

**Fig. 34**

**T3**                                          **pT3**

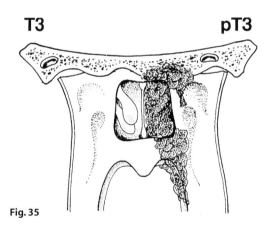

**Fig. 35**

**T4**                    **pT4**

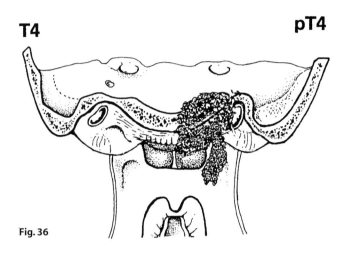

Fig. 36

**T4**                    **pT4**

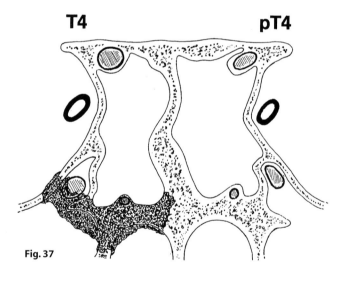

Fig. 37

## Hypopharynx

T1    Tumour limited to one subsite of hypopharynx (see p. 23) and 2 cm or less in greatest dimension (Figs. 38–40)

T2    Tumour invades more than one subsite of hypopharynx or an adjacent site, or measures more than 2 cm but not more than 4 cm in greatest dimension, *without* fixation of hemilarynx (Figs. 41–45)

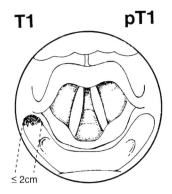

**Fig. 38.**    Involvement of the piriform sinus (C12.9)

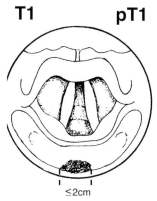

**Fig. 39.**    Involvement of the posterior wall (C13.2)

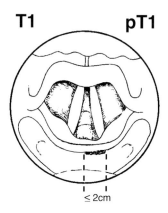

**Fig. 40.**    Involvement of the post-cricoid area (C13.0)

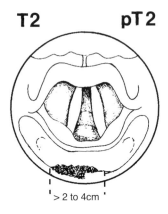

**Fig. 41.** Involvement of the posterior wall of the hypopharynx (C 13.2)

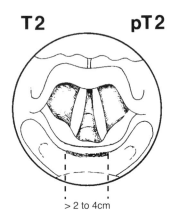

**Fig. 42.** Involvement of the postcricoid area (C13.0)

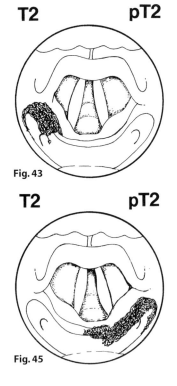

Fig. 43

Fig. 45

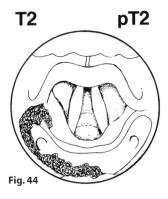

Fig. 44

**Fig. 43.** Involvement of the piriform sinus (C12.9) and the aryepiglottic fold (C13.1)

**Fig. 44.** Involvement of the piriform sinus (C12.9) and the posterior wall (C13.2)

**Fig. 45.** Involvement of the piriform sinus (C12.9) and the postcricoid area (C13.0)

T3    Tumour measures more than 4 cm in greatest dimension, or *with* fixation of hemilarynx (Figs. 46–48)

T4    Tumour invades adjacent structures, e.g. thyroid/cricoid cartilage, carotid artery, soft tissues of neck, prevertebral fascia/muscles, thyroid and/or oesophagus (Figs. 49, 50)

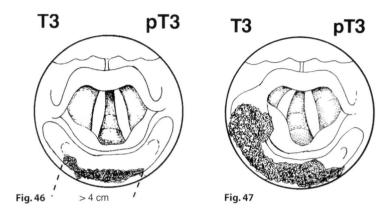

**T3**    **pT3**    **T3**    **pT3**

**Fig. 46** ·    > 4 cm    **Fig. 47**

**Fig. 46.** Involvement of the posterior wall (C13.2)

**Fig. 47.** Invasion of the piriform sinus (C12.9), the aryepiglottic fold (C13.1) and the posterior wall (C13.2) with fixation of the hemilarynx.

**Fig. 48.** Invasion of the piriform sinus (C12.9) and postcricoid area (C13.0) with fixation of the hemilarynx

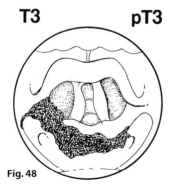

**T3**    **pT3**

**Fig. 48**

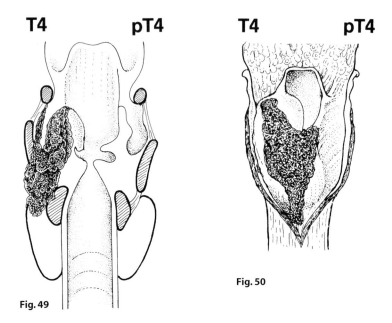

**Fig. 49**

**Fig. 50**

**Fig. 49.**   Invasion of the piriform sinus involving the thyroid and cricoid cartilage
**Fig. 50.**   Invasion of the postcricoid area involving the adjacent cervical oesophagus (not only mucosa but also deeper layers)

## N – Regional Lymph Nodes

*Oropharynx and Hypopharynx*
See p. 7.

*Nasopharynx*

NX    Regional lymph nodes cannot be assessed
N0    No regional lymph node metastasis

N1     Unilateral metastasis in lymph node(s), 6 cm or less in greatest dimen-
       sion, above supraclavicular fossa (Fig. 51)

**Note:**     Midline nodes are considered ipsilateral nodes.

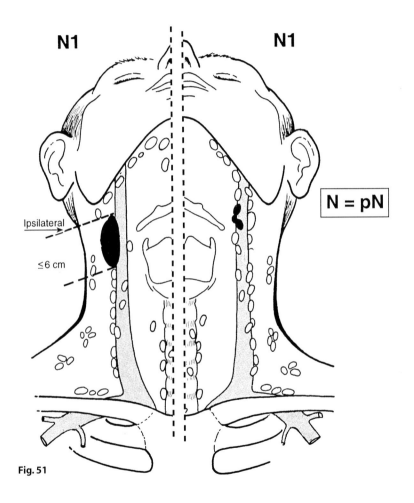

**Fig. 51**

N2    Bilateral metastasis in lymph node(s), 6 cm or less in greatest dimension, above supraclavicular fossa (Fig. 52)

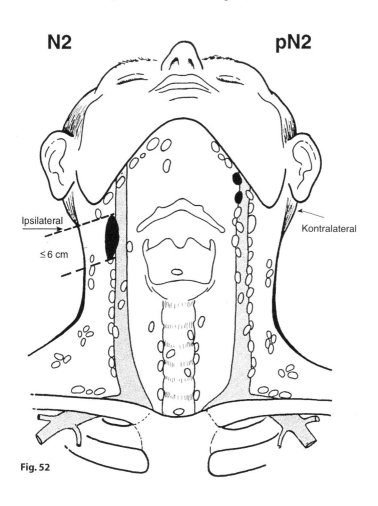

**Fig. 52**

N3    Metastasis in lymph node(s)
      (a) greater than 6 cm in dimension (Fig. 53)
      (b) in the supraclavicular fossa (Fig. 53)

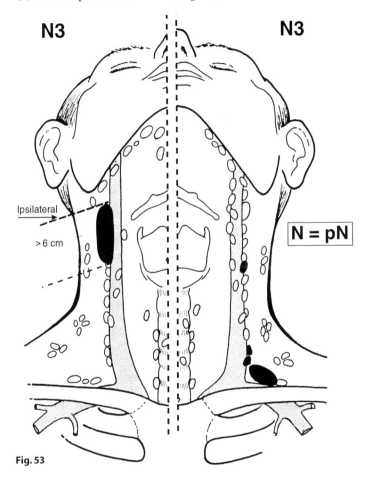

**Fig. 53**

## pTN Pathological Classification

The pT and pN categories correspond to the T and N categories.

pN0   Histological examination of a selective neck dissection specimen will
      ordinarily include 6 or more lymph nodes. Histological examination of a
      radical or modified radical neck dissection specimen will ordinarily
      include 10 or more lymph nodes.

# Larynx (ICD-O C32.0,1,2, C10.1)

## Rules for Classification

The classification applies only to carcinomas. There should be histological confirmation of the disease.

## Anatomical Sites and Subsites (Figs. 25, 26 [see p. 23], 54, 55)

**1. Supraglottis** (C32.1)
- i) Suprahyoid epiglottis [including tip, lingual (anterior) (C10.1) and laryngeal surfaces]
- ii) Aryepiglottic fold, laryngeal aspect
- iii) Arytenoid

Epilarynx (including marginal zone)

- iv) Infrahyoid epiglottis
- v) Ventricular bands (false cords)

Supraglottis excluding epilarynx

**2. Glottis** (C32.0)
- i) Vocal cords
- ii) Anterior commissure
- iii) Posterior commissure

**3. Subglottis** (C32.2)

## Regional Lymph Nodes

See p. 7.

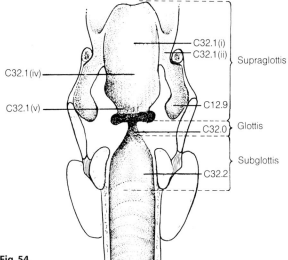

**Fig. 54**

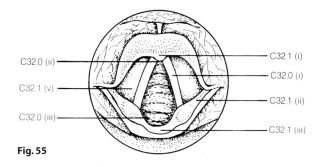

**Fig. 55**

# TN Clinical Classification

## T – Primary Tumour

TX   Primary tumour cannot be assessed
T0   No evidence of primary tumour
Tis  Carcinoma in situ

## *Supraglottis*

T1    Tumour limited to one subsite of supraglottis with normal vocal cord
      mobility (Figs. 56, 57)

**T1**

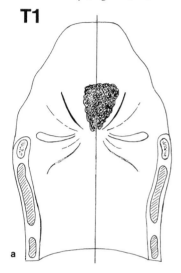

**pT1**

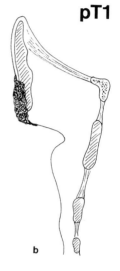

a                                                           b

**Fig. 56a, b.** Involvement of the epiglottis

**T1**

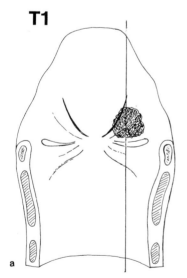

**pT1**

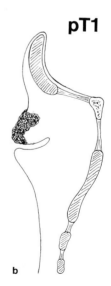

a                                                           b

**Fig. 57a, b.** Involvement of the false cord

T2    Tumour invades mucosa of more than one adjacent subsite of supraglot-
      tis or glottis or region outside the supraglottis (e.g. mucosa of base of
      tongue, vallecula, medial wall of piriform sinus) without fixation of the
      larynx (Figs. 58, 59)

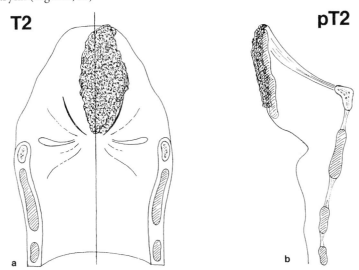

**Fig. 58a, b.** Involvement of the suprahyoid and the mucosa of the infrahyoid epiglottis

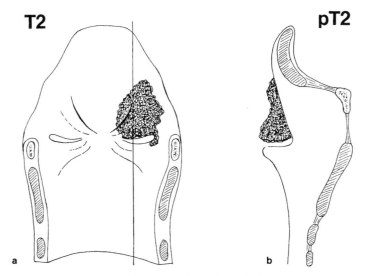

**Fig. 59a, b.** Involvement of the false cord and the epiglottis

T3    Tumour limited to larynx with vocal cord fixation and/or invades post-cricoid area and/or pre-epiglottic tissues (Figs. 60, 61)

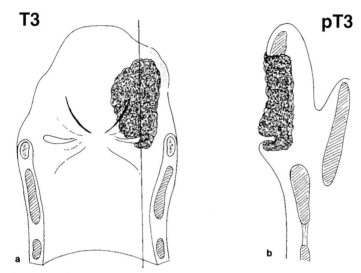

**Fig. 60.** Involvement of supraglottis and vocal cord with vocal cord fixation

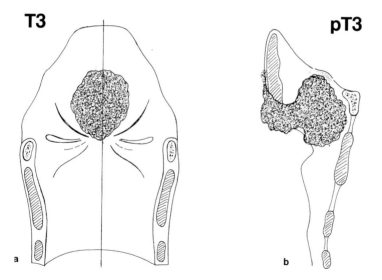

**Fig. 61.** Invasion of the pre-epiglottic tissues with vocal cord fixation

T4    Tumour invades through thyroid cartilage and/or extends into soft tissues of the neck, thyroid and/or oesophagus (Fig. 62)

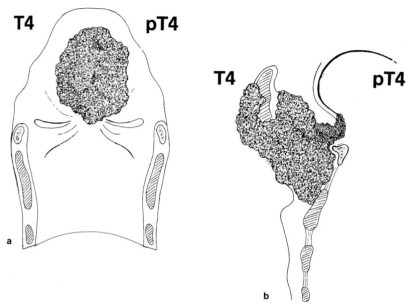

**Fig. 62.** Invasion beyond the larynx: oropharynx (vallecula and base of the tongue) and soft tissues of the neck (prelarynx)

## *Glottis*

T1    Tumour limited to vocal cord(s) (may involve anterior or posterior commissures) with normal mobility (Fig. 63a)

    T1a    Tumour limited to one vocal cord (Fig. 63b)

    T1b    Tumour involves both vocal cords (Fig. 63c)

T2    Tumour extends to supraglottis and/or subglottis, and/or with impaired vocal cord mobility (Fig. 64)

T3    Tumour limited to the larynx with vocal cord fixation (Fig. 65)

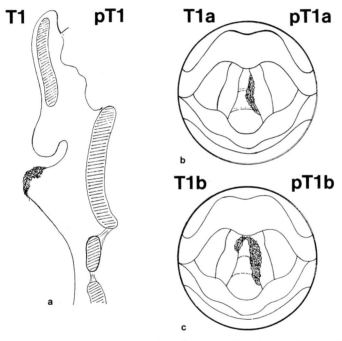

**Fig. 63a, b.** Tumour limited to vocal cord. **c** Tumour limited to vocal cords with invasion of the anterior commissure

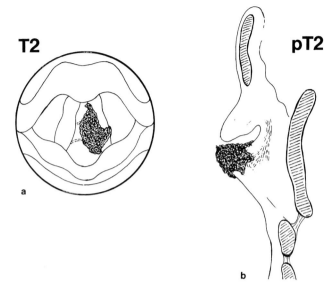

**Fig. 64a, b.** Tumour extends to supraglottis with impaired vocal cord mobility by invasion of the superficial m. vocalis

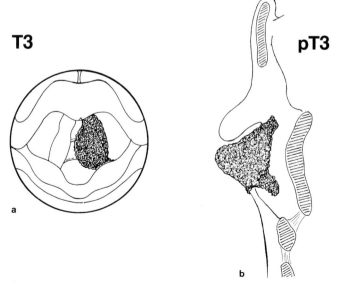

**Fig. 65a, b.** Tumour with vocal cord fixation

T4     Tumour invades through thyroid cartilage and/or extends to other tissues beyond the larynx, e.g. to trachea, soft tissues of the neck, thyroid, pharynx (Fig. 66)

**T4**

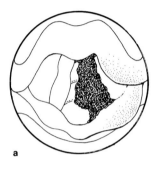

**pT4**

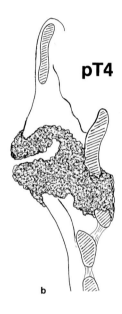

**Fig. 66a, b**

b

## Subglottis

T1    Tumour limited to subglottis (Fig. 67)
T2    Tumour extends to vocal cord(s) with normal or impaired mobility
        (Fig. 68)

**T1**

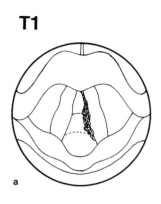

a

**Fig. 67a, b**

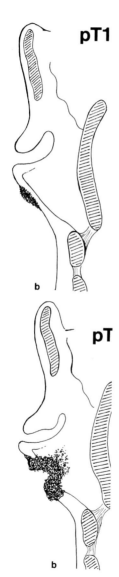

**pT1**

b

**T2**

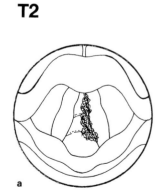

a

**Fig. 68a, b**

**pT**

b

T3    Tumour limited to larynx with vocal cord fixation (Fig. 69)
T4    Tumour invades through cricoid or thyroid cartilage and/or extends to other tissues beyond the larynx, e.g. trachea, soft tissues of the neck, thyroid, oesophagus (Fig. 70)

**T3**

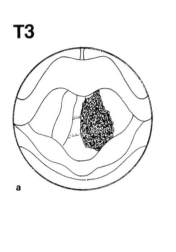

a

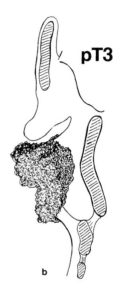

**pT3**

b

**Fig. 69a, b.**  Tumour with vocal cord fixation

**T4**

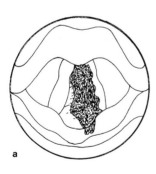

a

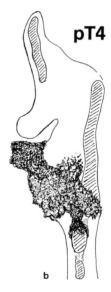

**pT4**

b

**Fig. 70a, b**

## N – Regional Lymph Nodes

See p. 7.

# pTN Pathological Classification

The pT and pN categories correspond to the T and N categories.

# Paranasal Sinuses (ICD-O C31.0,1)

## Rules for Classification

The classification applies only to carcinomas. There should be histological confirmation of the disease.

## Anatomical Subsites

1. Maxillary sinus (ICD-0 C31.0)
2. Ethmoid sinus (ICD-0 C31.1)

## Regional Lymph Nodes

See p. 7.

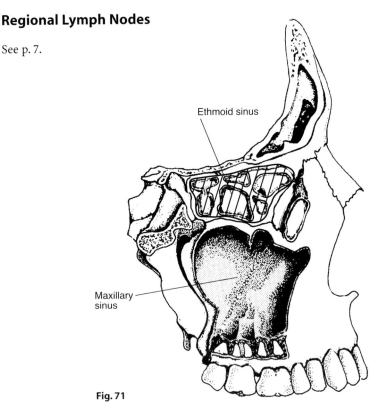

Ethmoid sinus

Maxillary sinus

**Fig. 71**

## TN Clinical Classification

### T – Primary Tumour

TX    Primary tumour cannot be assessed
T0    No evidence of primary tumour
Tis   Carcinoma in situ

#### Maxillary Sinus

T1    Tumour limited to the antral mucosa with no erosion or destruction of bone (Fig. 72)
T2    Tumour causing bone erosion or destruction, except for the posterior antral wall, including extension into hard palate and/or middle nasal meatus (Fig. 73)

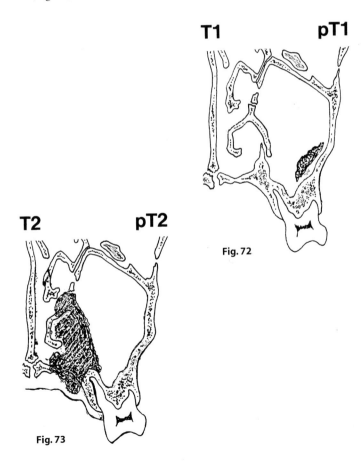

Fig. 72

Fig. 73

T3    Tumour invades any of the following: bone of posterior wall of maxillary sinus, subcutaneous tissues, skin of cheek, floor or medial wall of orbit, infratemporal fossa, pterygoid plates, ethmoid sinuses (Figs. 74, 75)

**T3**                    **T3**

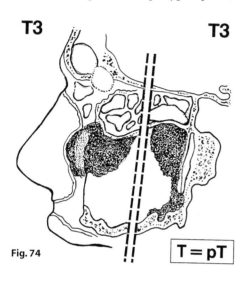

Fig. 74                    T = pT

**T3**              **T3**

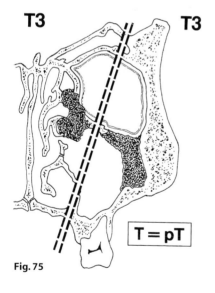

T = pT

Fig. 75

T4    Tumour invades orbital contents beyond the floor or medial wall including apex and/or any of the following: cribriform plate, base of skull, nasopharynx, sphenoid sinus, frontal sinus (Figs. 76–78)

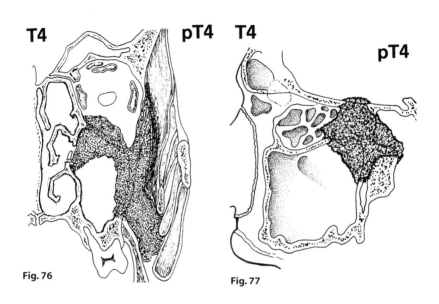

**T4**      **pT4**     **T4**

**pT4**

**Fig. 76**

**Fig. 77**

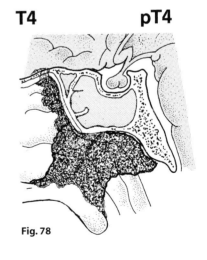

**T4**      **pT4**

**Fig. 78**

## Ethmoid Sinus

T1    Tumour confined to ethmoid with or without bone erosion (Fig. 79)
T2    Tumour extends into nasal cavitiy (Fig. 80)

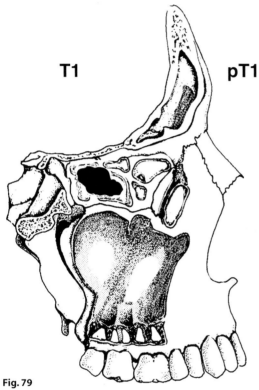

**T1**                              **pT1**

**Fig. 79**

**T2**

**pT2**

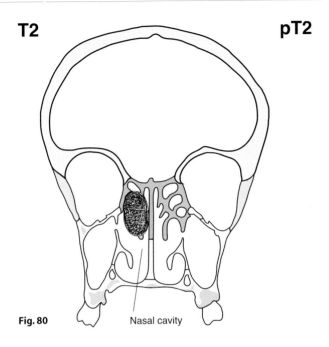

**Fig. 80**

Nasal cavity

T3    Tumour extends to anterior orbit and/or maxillary sinus (Fig. 81)
T4    Tumour with intracranial extension, orbital extension including apex, involving sphenoid and/or frontal sinus and/or skin of nose (Figs. 82, 83)

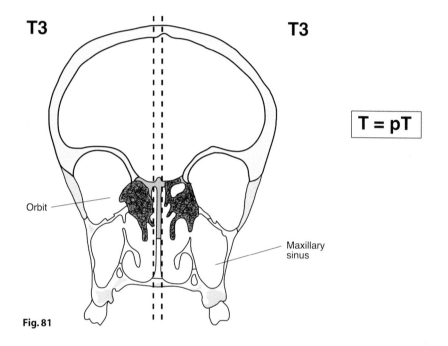

**T3**                                          **T3**

Orbit

Maxillary
sinus

T = pT

**Fig. 81**

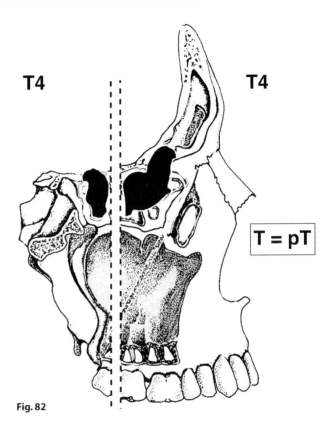

T4

T4

T = pT

**Fig. 82**

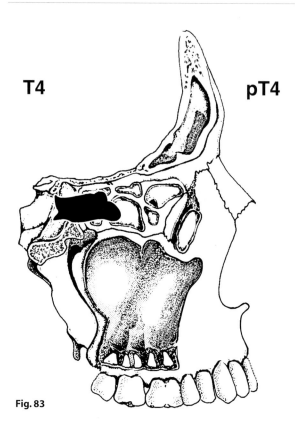

**T4**    **pT4**

**Fig. 83**

## N – Regional Lymph Nodes

See p. 7.

## pTN Pathological Classification

The pT and pN categories correspond to the T and N categories.

# Salivary Glands (ICD-O C07, C08)

## Rules for Classification

The classification applies only to carcinomas of the major salivary glands: parotid (C07.9), submandibular (submaxillary) (C08.0), and sublingual (C08.1) glands. Tumours arising in minor salivary glands (mucus-secreting glands in the lining membrane of the upper aerodigestive tract) are not included in this classification but at their anatomic site of origin, e.g. lip. There should be histological confirmation of the disease.

## Regional Lymph Nodes

See p. 7.

## TN Clinical Classification

### T – Primary Tumour

TX    Primary tumour cannot be assessed
T0    No evidence of primary tumour

T1    Tumour 2 cm or less in greatest dimension without extraparenchymal extension[1] (Fig. 84)
T2    Tumour more than 2 cm but not more than 4 cm in greatest dimension without extraparenchymal extension[1] (Fig. 85)

**Note:** 1. Extraparenchymal extension is clinical or macroscopic evidence of invasion of skin, soft tissues, bone, or nerve.
Microscopic evidence alone does not constitute extraparenchymal extension for classification purposes.

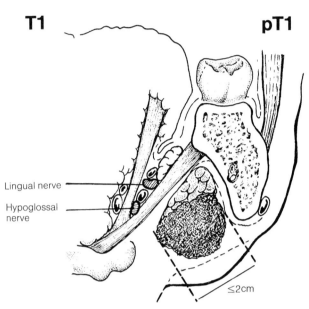

**T1**

**pT1**

Lingual nerve

Hypoglossal
nerve

≤2cm

**Fig. 84.** Classification determined clinically on the basis of absence of paralysis or macroscopically on the basis of no extraparenchymal extension. Frontal section through the premolar region

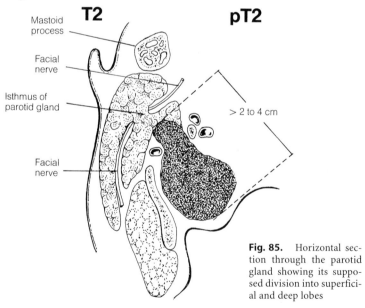

**T2**

**pT2**

Mastoid
process

Facial
nerve

Isthmus of
parotid gland

Facial
nerve

> 2 to 4 cm

**Fig. 85.** Horizontal section through the parotid gland showing its supposed division into superficial and deep lobes

T3    Tumour having extraparenchymal extension[1] without seventh nerve involvement and/or more than 4 cm but not more than 6 cm in greatest dimension (Figs. 86, 87)

**Note:**    1. See note p. 59.

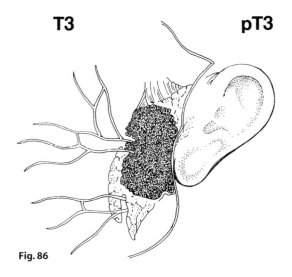

**T3**                                **pT3**

**Fig. 86**

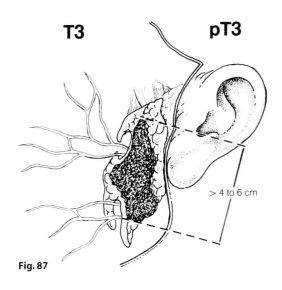

**T3**                                **pT3**

> 4 to 6 cm

**Fig. 87**

T4    Tumour invades base of skull, seventh nerve, and/or exceeds 6 cm in greatest dimension (Figs. 88, 89)

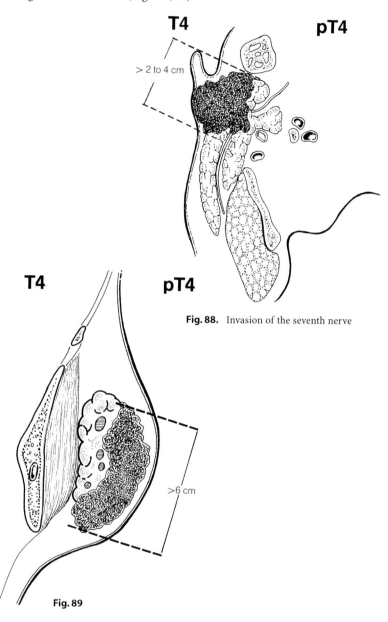

**Fig. 88.**   Invasion of the seventh nerve

**Fig. 89**

## N – Regional Lymph Nodes

See p. 7.

# pTN Pathological Classification

The pT and pN categories correspond to the T and N categories.

# Thyroid Gland (ICD-O C73) (Fig. 90)

## Rules for Classification

The classification applies only to carcinomas. There should be histological confirmation of the disease and division of cases by histological type.

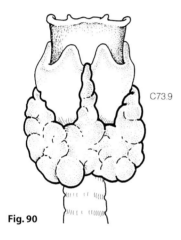

C73.9

**Fig. 90**

## Regional Lymph Nodes (Fig. 91)

The regional lymph nodes are the cervical (1) and upper mediastinal nodes (2).

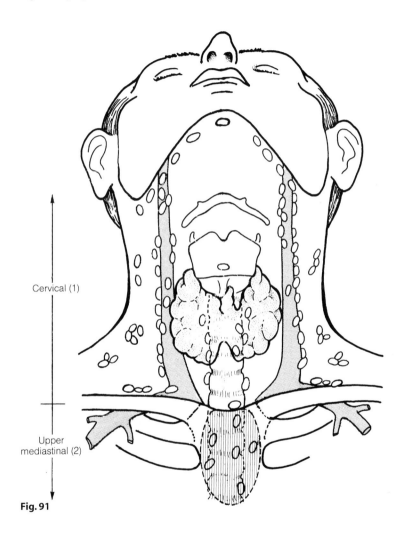

**Fig. 91**

## TN Clinical Classification

### T – Primary Tumour

TX    Primary tumour cannot be assessed
T0    No evidence of primary tumour

T1    Tumour 1 cm or less in greatest dimension, limited to the thyroid
      (Figs. 92, 93)
T2    Tumour more than 1 cm but not more than 4 cm in greatest dimension,
      limited to the thyroid (Figs. 94, 95)
T3    Tumour more than 4 cm in greatest dimension, limited to the thyroid
      (Fig. 96)
T4    Tumour of any size extending beyond the thyroid capsule (Fig. 97)

**Note:**  All categories may be subdivided: (a)solitary tumour (Figs. 92, 94, 96, 97);
      (b) multifocal tumour (the largest determines the classification) (Figs. 93, 95).

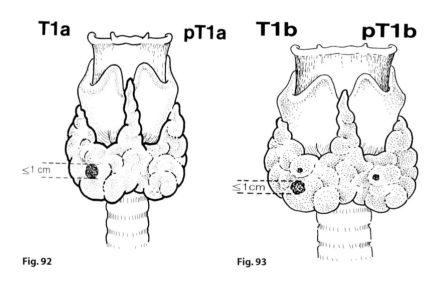

Fig. 92                          Fig. 93

**T2a    pT2a**

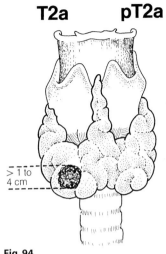

Fig. 94

**T2b    pT2b**

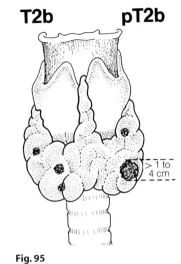

Fig. 95

**T3a    pT3a**

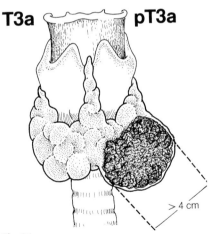

Fig. 96

**T4a    pT4a**

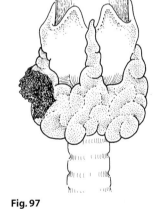

Fig. 97

## N – Regional Lymph Nodes

NX    Regional lymph nodes cannot be assessed
N0    No regional lymph node metastasis
N1    Regional lymph node metastasis
    N1a    Metastasis in ipsilateral cervical lymph node(s) (Fig. 98)
    N1b    Metastasis in bilateral (Fig. 99), midline (Fig. 100) or contralateral
        cervical (Fig. 101) or mediastinal lymph node(s) (Fig. 102)

## pTN Pathological Classification

The pT and pN categories correspond to the T and N categories.

pN0    Histological examination of a selective neck dissection specimen will
    ordinarily include 6 or more lymph nodes.

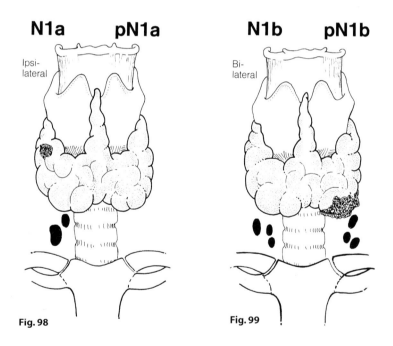

**N1a**    **pN1a**    **N1b**    **pN1b**

Ipsi-
lateral

Bi-
lateral

**Fig. 98**    **Fig. 99**

**N1b**    **pN1b**

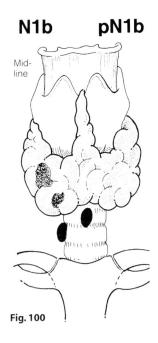

Mid-
line

**Fig. 100**

**N1b**    **pN1b**

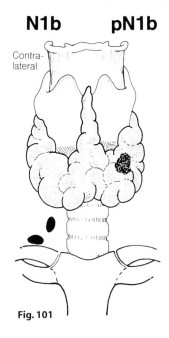

Contra-
lateral

**Fig. 101**

**N1b**    **pN1b**

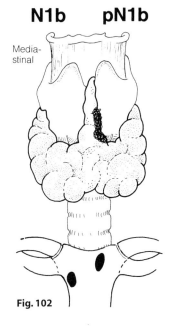

Media-
stinal

**Fig. 102**

# Digestive System Tumours

## Introductory Notes

The following sites are included:

| | |
|---|---|
| Oesophagus | Liver |
| Stomach | Gallbladder |
| Small intestine | Extrahepatic bile ducts |
| Colon and rectum | Ampulla of Vater |
| Anal canal | Pancreas (excluding endocrine) |

## Regional Lymph Nodes

The number of lymph nodes ordinarily included in a lymphadenectomy specimen is noted at each site. The designation pN0 is usually based on this figure.

## Oesophagus (ICD-O C15)

### Rules for Classification

The classification applies only to carcinomas. There should be histological confirmation of the disease and division of cases by histological type.

### Anatomical Subsites (Fig. 103)

1. Cervical oesophagus (C15.0): This commences at the lower border of the cricoid cartilage and ends at the thoracic inlet (suprasternal notch), approximately 18 cm from the upper incisor teeth
2. Intrathoracic oesophagus
   i)   The upper thoracic portion (C15.3) extending from the thoracic inlet to the level of the tracheal bifurcation, approximately 24 cm from the upper incisor teeth
   ii)  The mid-thoracic portion (C15.4) is the proximal half of the oesophagus between the tracheal bifurcation and the oesophagogastric junction. The lower level is approximately 32 cm from the upper incisor teeth
   iii) The lower thoracic portion (C15.5), approximately 8 cm in length (includes abdominal oesophagus), is the distal half of the oesophagus between the tracheal bifurcation and the oesophagogastric junction. The lower level is approximately 40 cm from the upper incisor teeth

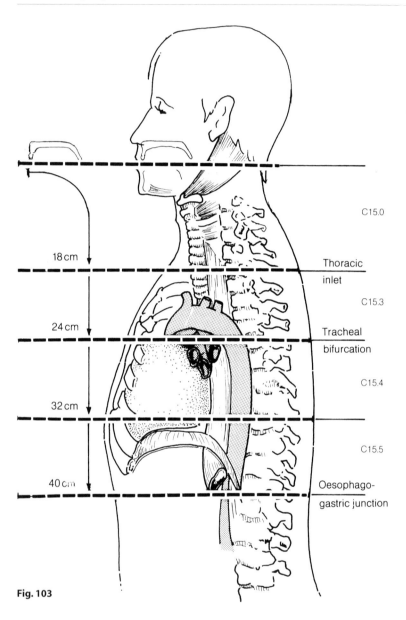

18 cm

24 cm

32 cm

40 cm

C15.0

Thoracic
inlet

C15.3

Tracheal
bifurcation

C15.4

C15.5

Oesophago-
gastric junction

**Fig. 103**

## Regional Lymph Nodes (Fig. 104)

The regional lymph nodes are, for the cervical oesophagus, the cervical nodes including supraclavicular nodes and, for the intrathoracic oesophagus, the mediastinal and perigastric nodes, excluding the coeliac nodes.

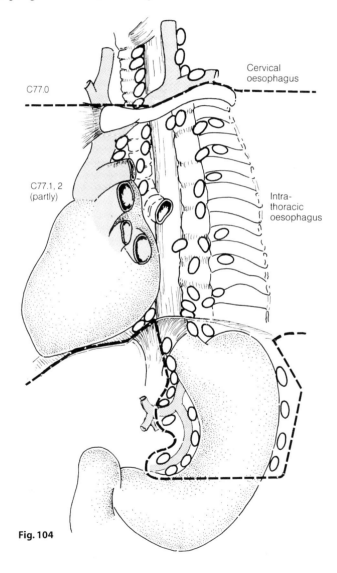

C77.0

Cervical oesophagus

C77.1, 2 (partly)

Intra-thoracic oesophagus

**Fig. 104**

## TNM Clinical Classification

### T – Primary Tumour

TX    Primary tumour cannot be assessed
T0    No evidence of primary tumour
Tis   Carcinoma in situ

T1    Tumour invades lamina propria or submucosa (Fig. 105)
T2    Tumour invades muscularis propria (Fig. 106)

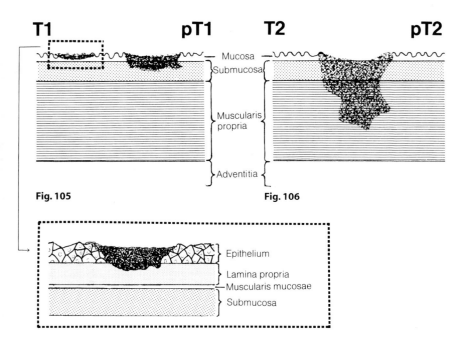

**Fig. 105**    **Fig. 106**

T3    Tumour invades adventitia (Fig. 107)
T4    Tumour invades adjacent structures (Fig. 108)

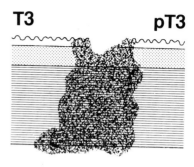

Fig. 107

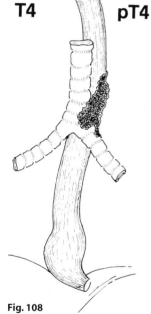

Fig. 108

## N – Regional Lymph Nodes

NX    Regional lymph nodes cannot be assessed
N0    No regional lymph node metastasis
N1    Regional lymph node metastasis (Figs. 109–112)

# Carcinoma of cervical oesophagus

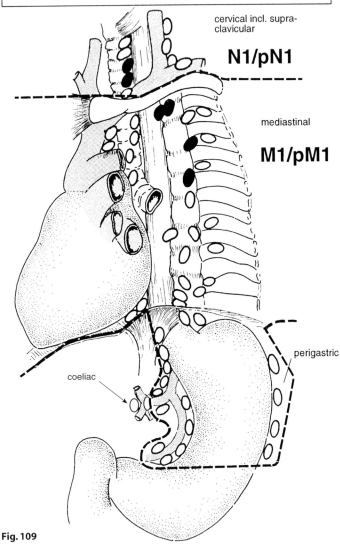

cervical incl. supra-
clavicular

**N1/pN1**

mediastinal

**M1/pM1**

perigastric

coeliac

**Fig. 109**

# Carcinoma of upper thoracic oesophagus

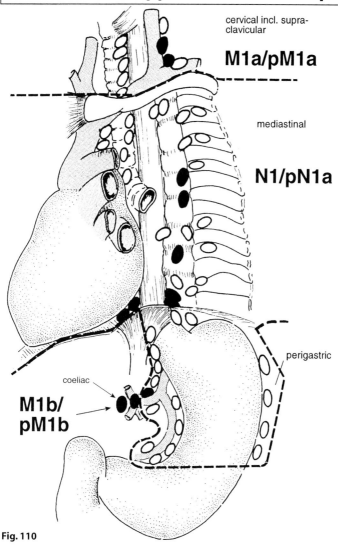

cervical incl. supra-
clavicular

**M1a/pM1a**

mediastinal

**N1/pN1a**

perigastric

coeliac

**M1b/
pM1b**

Fig. 110

## Carcinoma of mid-thoracic oesophagus

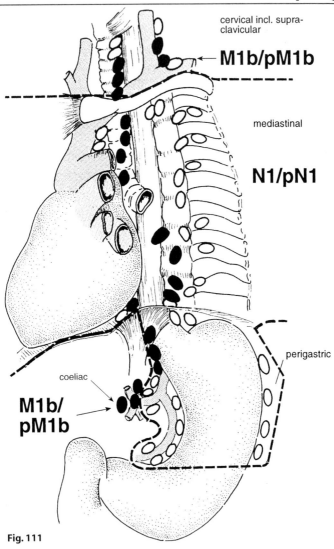

cervical incl. supra-clavicular

**M1b/pM1b**

mediastinal

**N1/pN1**

perigastric

coeliac

**M1b/ pM1b**

Fig. 111

# Carcinoma of lower thoracic oesophagus

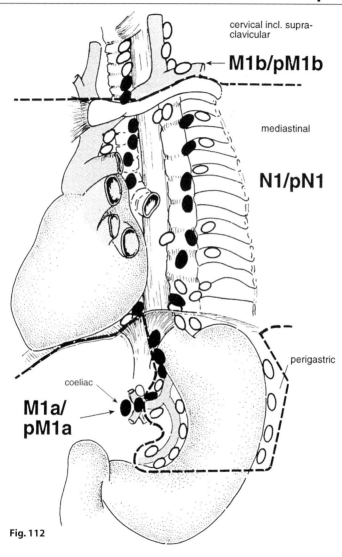

cervical incl. supra-
clavicular

**M1b/pM1b**

mediastinal

**N1/pN1**

perigastric

coeliac

**M1a/
pM1a**

**Fig. 112**

## M – Distant Metastasis

MX  Distant metastasis cannot be assessed
M0  No distant metastasis
M1  Distant metastasis (Figs. 109–112)

**For tumours of lower thoracic oesophagus**
M1a  Metastasis in coeliac lymph nodes
M1b  Other distant metastasis

**For tumours of upper thoracic oesophagus**
M1a  Metastasis in cervical lymph nodes
M1b  Other distant metastasis

**For tumours of mid-thoracic oesophagus**
M1a  Not applicable
M1b  Non-regional lymph node or other distant metastasis

# pTNM Pathological Classification

The pT, pN and pM categories correspond to the T, N and M categories.

pN0  Histological examination of a mediastinal lymphadenectomy specimen
     will ordinarily include 6 or more lymph nodes.

# Stomach (ICD-O C16)

## Rules for Classification

The classification applies only to carcinomas. There should be histological confirmation of the disease.

## Anatomical Subsites (Fig. 113)

1. Cardia (C16.0)
2. Fundus (C16.1)
3. Corpus (C16.2)
4. Antrum (C16.3) and pylorus (C16.4)

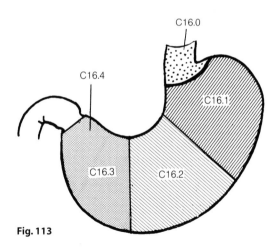

**Fig. 113**

## Regional Lymph Nodes (Fig. 114)

The regional lymph nodes are the perigastric nodes along the lesser (1, 3, 5) and greater (2, 4a, 4b, 6) curvatures, the nodes located along the left gastric (7), common hepatic (8), splenic (10, 11) and coeliac arteries (9) and the hepatoduodenal nodes (12). Involvement of other intra-abdominal lymph nodes such as the retropancreatic, mesenteric and para-aortic is classified as distant metastasis.

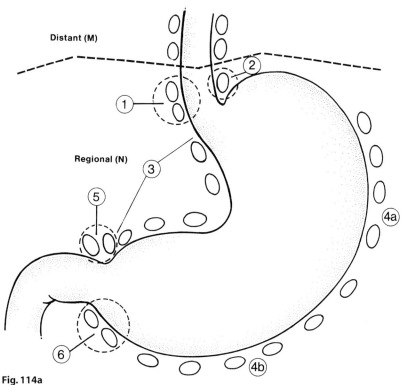

Fig. 114a

**Note:** The numerical order corresponds to the proposals of the Japanese Research Society for Gastric Cancer [(1995) *Japanese Classification of Gastric Carcinoma*, 1st English edn. Kanehara, Tokyo].

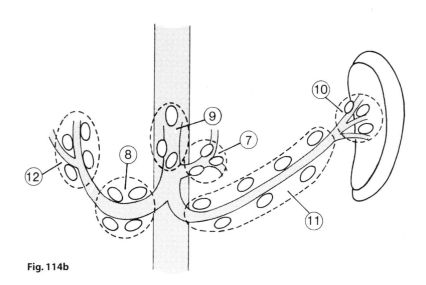

**Fig. 114b**

## TNM Clinical Classification

### T – Primary Tumour

TX    Primary tumour cannot be assessed
T0    No evidence of primary tumour
Tis   Carcinoma in situ: intraepithelial tumour without invasion of lamina propria

T1    Tumour invades lamina propria or submucosa (Fig. 115)
T2    Tumour invades muscularis propria or subserosa[1] (Figs. 116, 117)

**Note:** 1 see p. 87.

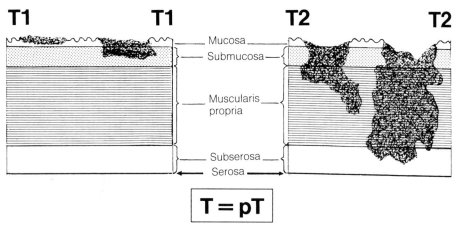

**Fig. 115**                                **Fig. 116**

# T2

# pT2

Serosa (visceral peritoneum)
Subserosa
Muscularis propria

Lesser
omentum

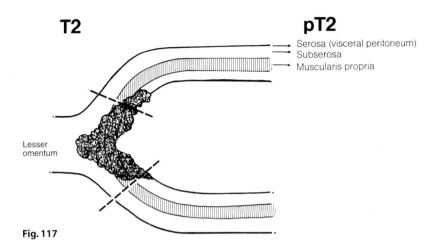

**Fig. 117**

T3    Tumour penetrates serosa (visceral peritoneum) without invasion of adjacent structures[1,2,3] (Figs. 118, 120)

T4    Tumour invades adjacent structures[1,2,3] (Fig. 119)

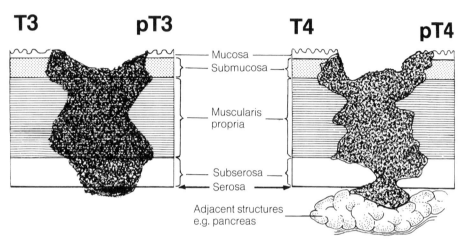

Fig. 118                                    Fig. 119

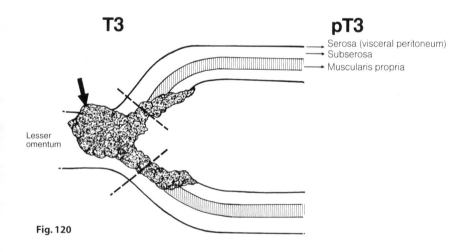

Fig. 120

**Notes:**  1. A tumour may penetrate the muscularis propria with extension into the gastrocolic or gastrohepatic ligaments or the greater or lesser omentum without perforation of the visceral peritoneum covering these structures. In this case, the tumour is classified as T2 (Fig. 117). If there is perforation of the visceral peritoneum covering the gastric ligaments or omenta, the tumour is classified as T3 (Fig. 120).

2. The adjacent structures of the stomach are the spleen, transverse colon, liver, diaphragm, pancreas, abdominal wall, adrenal gland, kidney, small intestine and retroperitoneum.

3. Intramural extension to the duodenum or oesophagus is classified by the depth of greatest invasion in any of these sites including stomach (Figs. 121, 122).

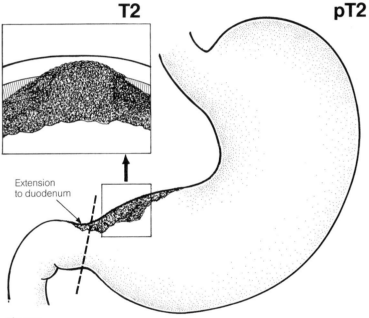

**T2**                                                    **pT2**

Extension
to duodenum

**Fig. 121**

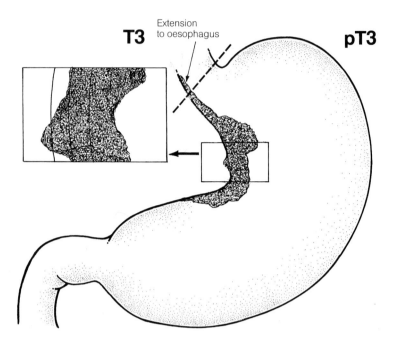

**T3**  Extension to oesophagus    **pT3**

**Fig. 122**

## N – Regional Lymph Nodes

NX    Regional lymph nodes cannot be assessed
N0    No regional lymph node metastasis
N1    Metastasis in 1 to 6 regional lymph nodes (Fig. 123)
N2    Metastasis in 7 to 15 regional lymph nodes (Fig. 124)
N3    Metastasis in more than 15 regional lymph nodes (Fig. 125)

N1

pN1

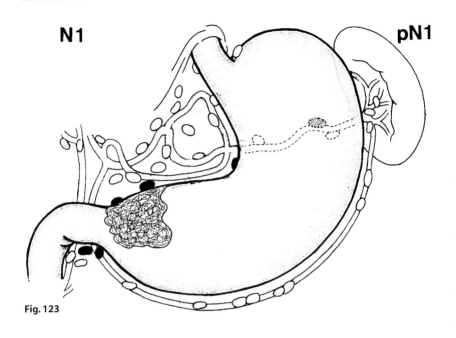

Fig. 123

N2

pN2

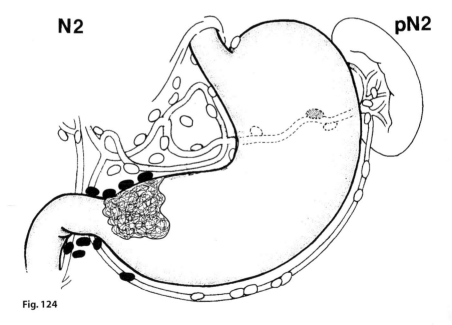

Fig. 124

**N3**

**pN3**

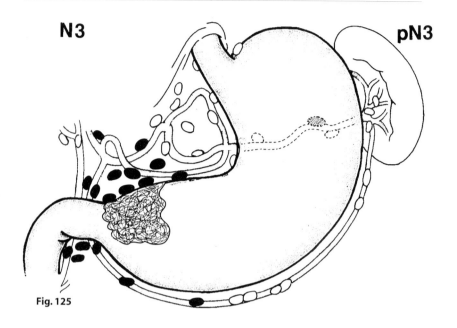

**Fig. 125**

## M – Distant Metastasis

MX    Distant metastasis cannot be assessed
M0    No distant metastasis
M1    Distant metastasis (Fig. 126)

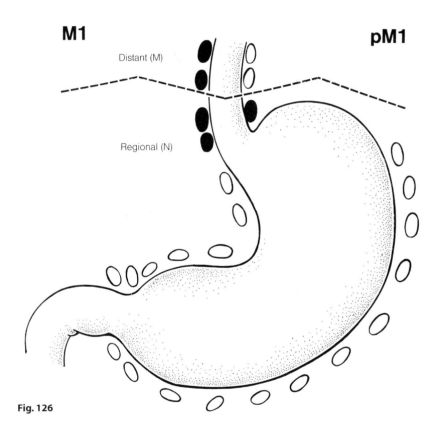

**M1**

**pM1**

Distant (M)

Regional (N)

**Fig. 126**

## pTNM Pathological Classification

The pT, pN and pM categories correspond to the T, N and M categories.

pN0    Histological examination of a regional lymphadenectomy specimen will ordinarily include 15 or more lymph nodes.

# Small Intestine (ICD-O C17)

## Rules for Classification

The classification applies only to carcinomas. There should be histological confirmation of the disease.

## Anatomical Sites (Fig. 127)

1. Duodenum (C17.0)
2. Jejunum (C17.1)
3. Ileum (C17.2) (excludes ileocecal valve C18.0)

**Note:** This classification does not apply to carcinomas of the ampulla of Vater (see p. 136).

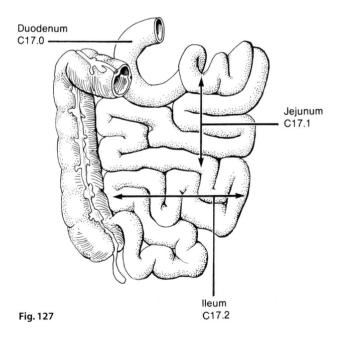

**Fig. 127**

## Regional Lymph Nodes

The regional lymph nodes for the duodenum (see Fig. 195, pp. 147) are the pancreaticoduodenal, pyloric, hepatic (pericholedochal, cystic, hilar) and superior mesenteric nodes.

The regional lymph nodes for the jejunum and ileum are the mesenteric nodes, including the superior mesenteric nodes, and, for the terminal ileum only, the ileocolic nodes including the posterior cecal nodes.

## TN Clinical Classification

### T – Primary Tumour

TX    Primary tumour cannot be assessed
T0    No evidence of primary tumour
Tis   Carcinoma in situ

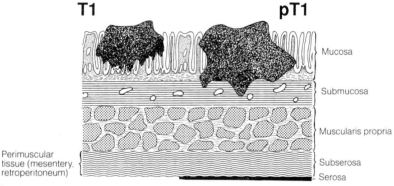

**Fig. 128**

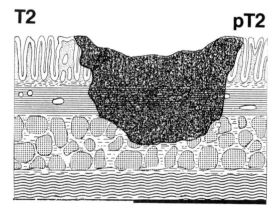

**Fig. 129**

T1    Tumour invades lamina propria or submucosa (Fig. 128)
T2    Tumour invades muscularis propria (Fig. 129)
T3    Tumour invades through muscularis propria into subserosa (Fig. 130) or into non-peritonealized perimuscular tissue (mesentery or retroperitoneum[1]) with extension 2 cm or less (Fig. 131)
T4    Tumour perforates visceral peritoneum (Fig. 130) or directly invades other organs or structures [includes other loops of small intestine (Fig. 132), mesentery or retroperitoneum more than 2 cm (Fig. 131), and abdonal wall by way of serosa; for duodenum only, invasion of pancreas (Fig. 133)]

**Note:**    1. The non-peritonealized perimuscular tissue is, for jejunum and ileum, part of the mesentery and, for duodenum in areas where serosa is lacking, part of the retroperitoneum.

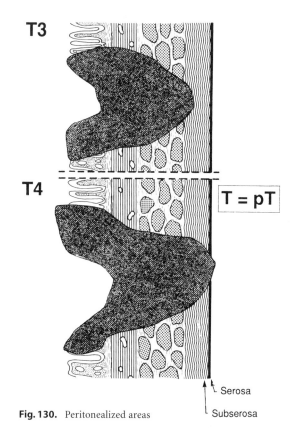

**Fig. 130.**   Peritonealized areas

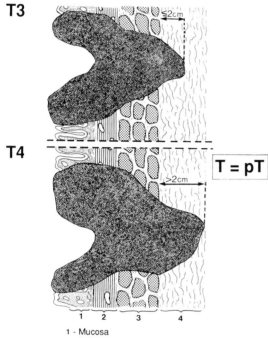

**T3**

**T4**

**T = pT**

1 - Mucosa
2 - Submucosa
3 - Muscularis propria
4 - Perimuscular
    tissue (mesentery,
    retroperitoneum)

**Fig. 131.** Non-peritonealized areas

**pT4**

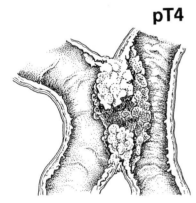

**Fig. 132**    **T4**

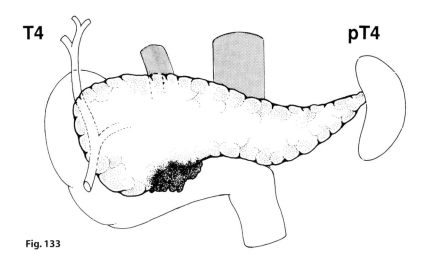

**T4**                                                                    **pT4**

**Fig. 133**

## N – Regional Lymph Nodes

NX    Regional lymph nodes cannot be assessed
N0    No regional lymph node metastasis
N1    Regional lymph node metastasis

## pTN Pathological Classification

The pT and pN categories correspond to the T and N categories.

pN0    Histological examination of a regional lymphadenectomy specimen will
          ordinarily include 6 or more lymph nodes.

# Colon and Rectum (ICD-O C18-C20)

## Rules for Classification

The classification applies only to carcinomas. There should be histological confirmation of the disease.

## Anatomical Sites and Subsites

*Colon* (Fig. 134)
1. Appendix (C18.1)
2. Cecum (C18.0)
3. Ascending colon (C18.2)
4. Hepatic flexure (C18.3)
5. Transverse colon (C18.4)
6. Splenic flexure (C18.5)
7. Descending colon (C18.6)
8. Sigmoid colon (C18.7)

*Rectum* (Fig. 135)
1. Rectosigmoid junction (C19.9)
2. Rectum (C20.9)

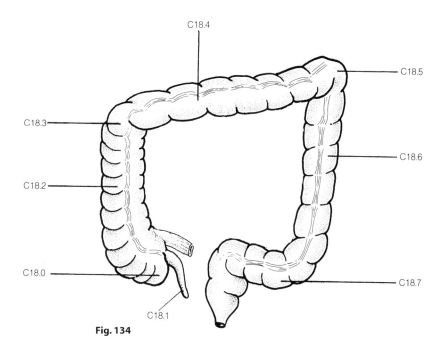

C18.4

C18.5

C18.3

C18.6

C18.2

C18.0

C18.7

C18.1

**Fig. 134**

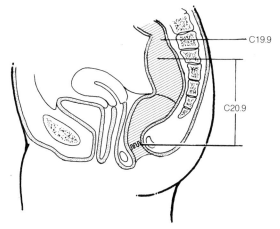

C19.9

C20.9

**Fig. 135**

## Regional Lymph Nodes (Fig. 136)

The regional lymph nodes are the pericolic and perirectal and those located along the ileocolic, right colic, middle colic, left colic, inferior mesenteric, superior rectal (haemorrhoidal) and internal iliac arteries (see Fig. 146, p. 108).

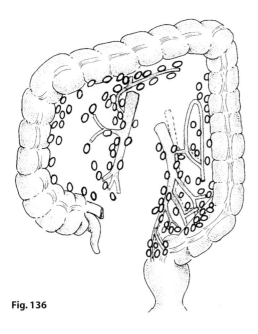

**Fig. 136**

# TN Clinical Classification

## T – Primary Tumour

TX    Primary tumour cannot be assessed
T0    No evidence of primary tumour
Tis   Carcinoma in situ: intraepithelial or invasion of lamina propria[1]

T1    Tumour invades submucosa (Fig. 137)
T2    Tumour invades muscularis propria (Fig. 138)

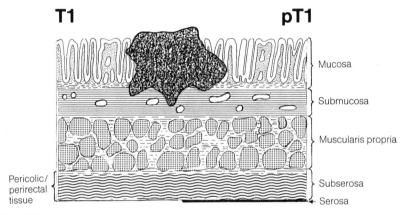

**Fig. 137**

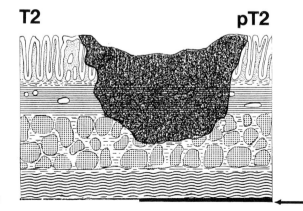

**Fig. 138**

T3    Tumour invades through muscularis propria into subserosa or into non-peritonealized pericolic or perirectal tissues (Fig. 139)

T4    Tumour directly invades other organs or structures[2] and/or perforates visceral peritoneum (Figs. 140, 141)

**Notes:**  1. Tis includes cancer cells confined within the glandular basement membrane (intraepithelial) or lamina propria (intramucosal) with no extension through the muscularis mucosae into the submucosa.

2. Direct invasion in T4 includes invasion of other segments of the colorectum by way of the serosa, e.g. invasion of the sigmoid colon by a carcinoma of the cecum.

**T3**                           **pT3**

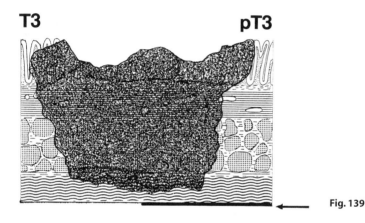

Fig. 139

**T4**                           **pT4**

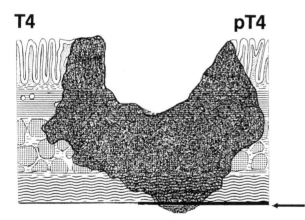

Fig. 140

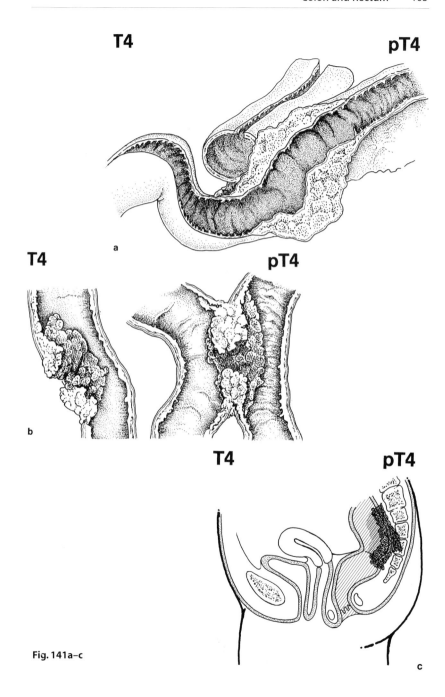

T4    pT4

T4    pT4

a

T4    pT4

b

T4    pT4

Fig. 141a–c

c

## N – Regional Lymph Nodes

NX    Regional lymph nodes cannot be assessed
N0    No regional lymph node metastasis
N1    Metastasis in 1 to 3 regional lymph nodes (Fig. 142)
N2    Metastasis in 4 or more regional lymph nodes (Figs. 143, 144)

**Note:**    A tumour nodule greater than 3 mm in diameter in perirectal or pericolic adipose tissue without histological evidence of a residual lymph node in the nodule is classified as regional lymph node metastasis. However, a tumour nodule up to 3 mm in diameter is classified in the T category as discontinuous extension, i.e. T3.

## pTN Pathological Classification

The pT and pN categories correspond to the T and N categories.

pN0    Histological examination of a regional lymphadenectomy specimen will ordinarily include 12 or more lymph nodes.

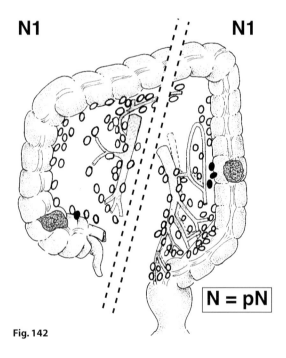

**N1**    **N1**

**N = pN**

**Fig. 142**

**N2**

**N2**

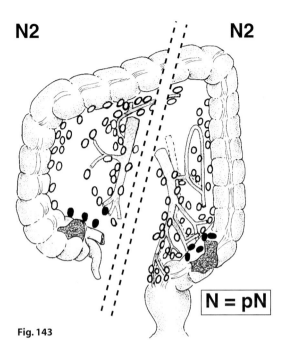

N = pN

**Fig. 143**

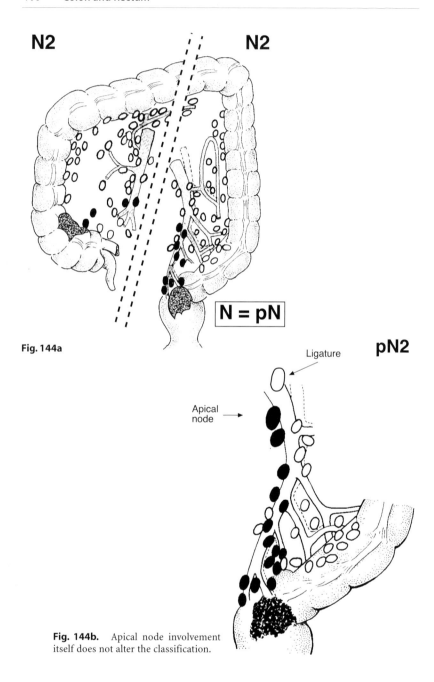

**N2**    **N2**

N = pN

**Fig. 144a**

pN2

Ligature

Apical
node

**Fig. 144b.**   Apical node involvement
itself does not alter the classification.

# Anal Canal (ICD-O C21.1,2)

The anal canal (Fig. 145) extends from the rectum to the perianal skin (to the junction with hair-bearing skin). It is lined by the mucous membrane overlying the internal sphincter, including the transitional epithelium and dentate line Tumours of the anal margin (ICD-O C44.5) are classified with skin tumours (p. 179).

## Rules for Classification

The classification applies only to carcinomas. There should be histological confirmation of the disease.

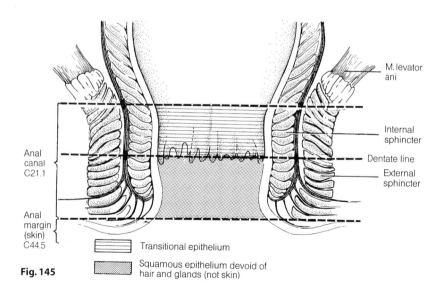

Anal canal C21.1

Anal margin (skin) C44.5

M. levator ani

Internal sphincter

Dentate line

External sphincter

Transitional epithelium

Squamous epithelium devoid of hair and glands (not skin)

**Fig. 145**

## Regional Lymph Nodes (Fig. 146)

The regional lymph nodes are the perirectal (1), the internal iliac (2) and the inguinal lymph nodes (3).

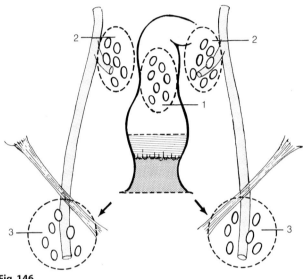

**Fig. 146**

## TN Clinical Classification

### T – Primary Tumour

TX   Primary tumour cannot be assessed
T0   No evidence of primary tumour
Tis  Carcinoma in situ

T1   Tumour 2 cm or less in greatest dimension (Fig. 147)
T2   Tumour more than 2 cm but not more than 5 cm in greatest dimension (Fig. 148)
T3   Tumour more than 5 cm in greatest dimension (Fig. 149)

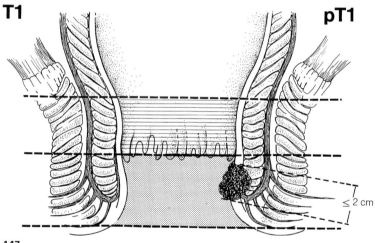

**Fig. 147**

**T2**

**T2**

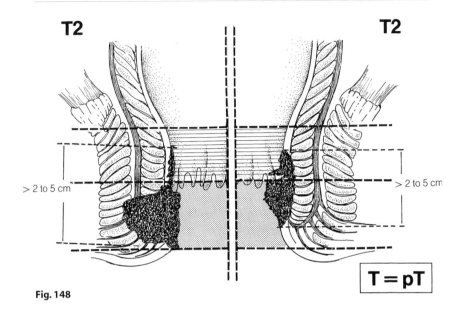

> 2 to 5 cm

> 2 to 5 cm

$$T = pT$$

**Fig. 148**

**T3**

**pT3**

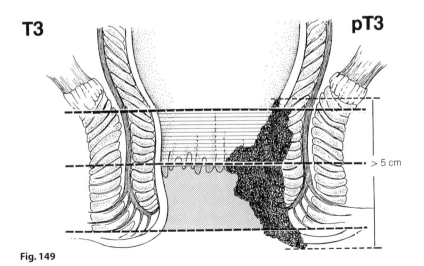

> 5 cm

**Fig. 149**

T4     Tumour of any size invades adjacent organ(s), e.g. vagina, urethra, bladder (Fig. 150) (involvement of the sphincter muscle(s) alone is not classified as T4)

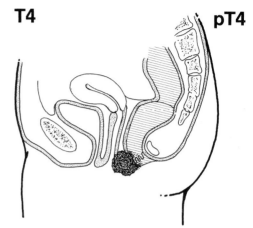

**Fig. 150**

## N – Regional Lymph Nodes

NX     Regional lymph nodes cannot be assessed
N0     No regional lymph node metastasis
N1     Metastasis in perirectal lymph node(s) (Fig. 151)

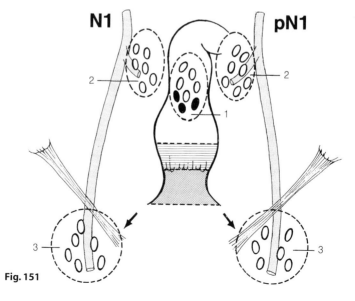

**Fig. 151**

N2    Metastasis in unilateral internal iliac and/or inguinal lymph node(s) (Figs. 152, 153)

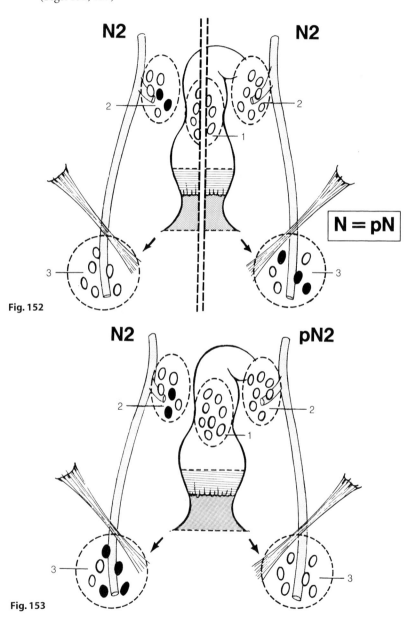

Fig. 152

Fig. 153

N3    Metastasis in perirectal and inguinal lymph nodes and/or bilateral internal iliac and/or inguinal lymph nodes (Figs. 154-156)

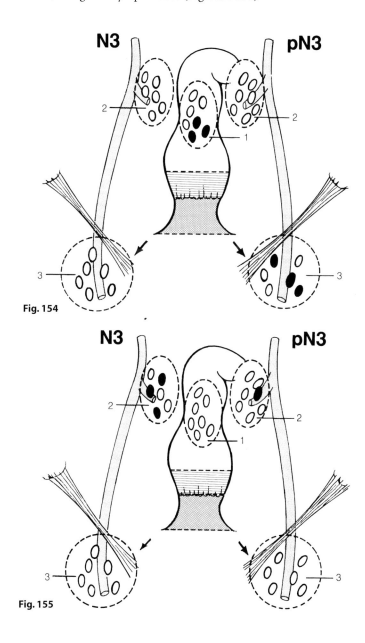

**Fig. 154**

**Fig. 155**

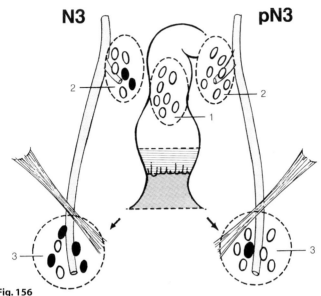

**Fig. 156**

## pTN Pathological Classification

The pT and pN categories correspond to the T and N categories.

pN0    Histological examination of a regional perirectal-pelvic lymphadenec-
       tomy specimen will ordinarily include 12 or more lymph nodes. Histo-
       logical examination of an inguinal lymphadenectomy specimen will
       ordinarily include 6 or more lymph nodes.

# Liver (ICD-O C22)

## Rules for Classification

The classification applies only to primary hepatocellular and cholangio- (intrahepatic bile duct) carcinoma of the liver. There should be histological confirmation of the disease and division of cases by histological type.

**Note:** Although the presence of cirrhosis is an important prognostic factor, it does not affect the TNM classification, being an independent variable.

## Anatomical Subsites (Fig. 157)

1. Liver (C22.0)
2. Intrahepatic bile duct (C22.1)

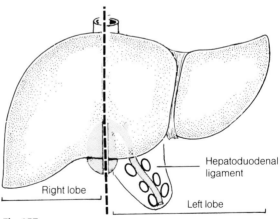

**Fig. 157**

## Regional Lymph Nodes (Fig. 157)

The regional lymph nodes are the hilar nodes (i.e. those in the hepatoduodenal ligament).

## TN Clinical Classification

### T – Primary Tumour

TX    Primary tumour cannot be assessed
T0    No evidence of primary tumour

T1    Solitary tumour 2 cm or less in greatest dimension without vascular invasion (Fig. 158)

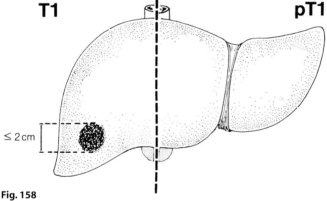

**Fig. 158**

T2    Solitary tumour 2 cm or less in greatest dimension with vascular invasion (Fig. 159);
*or* multiple tumours limited to one lobe, none more than 2 cm in greatest dimension without vascular invasion (Fig. 160);
*or* solitary tumour more than 2 cm in greatest dimension without vascular invasion (Fig. 161)

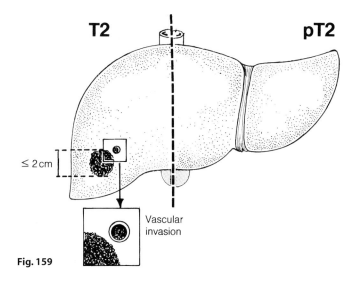

**Fig. 159**

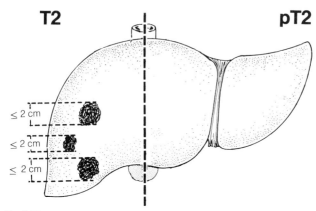

**Fig. 160**

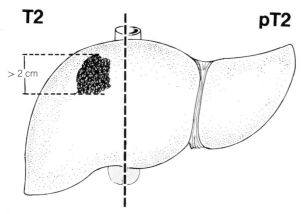

**Fig. 161**

T3    Solitary tumour more than 2 cm in greatest dimension with vascular invasion (Fig. 162);
or multiple tumours limited to one lobe, none more than 2 cm in greatest dimension with vascular invasion (Fig. 163);
or multiple tumours limited to one lobe, any more than 2 cm in greatest dimension with or without vascular invasion (Figs. 164, 165)

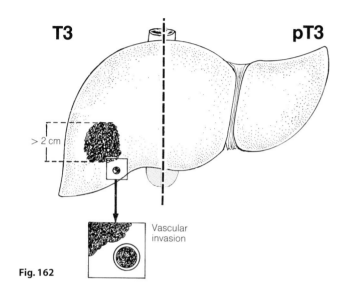

**T3**                    **pT3**

> 2 cm

Vascular
invasion

**Fig. 162**

Vascular
invasion

**T3**                    **pT3**

≤ 2 cm

≤ 2 cm

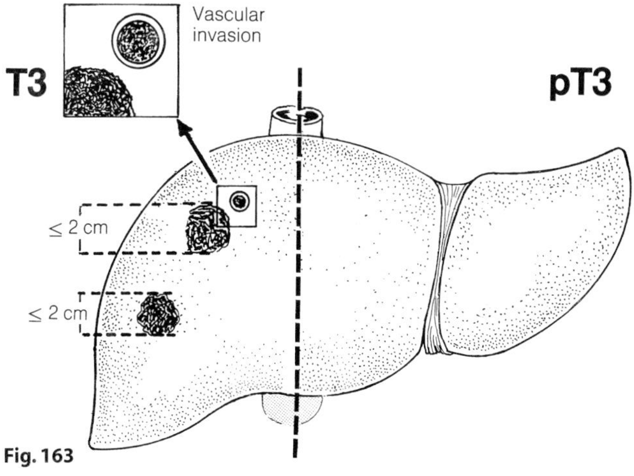

**Fig. 163**

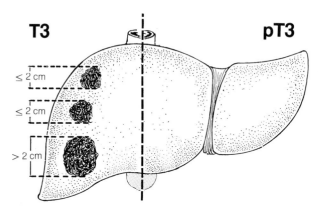

**T3**                    **pT3**

≤ 2 cm

≤ 2 cm

> 2 cm

**Fig. 164**

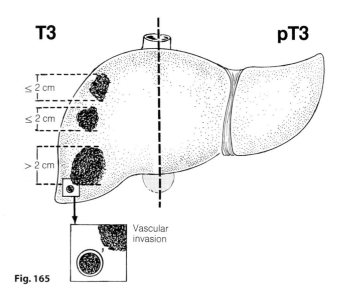

**T3**                    **pT3**

≤ 2 cm

≤ 2 cm

> 2 cm

Vascular
invasion

**Fig. 165**

T4    Multiple tumours in more than one lobe (Fig. 166)
      *or* tumour(s) involve(s) a major branch of the portal or hepatic vein(s) (Fig. 167);
      *or* tumour(s) with direct invasion of adjacent organs other than gall-bladder;
      *or* tumour(s) with perforation of visceral peritoneum (Fig. 168)

**Note:**    For classification, the plane projecting between the bed of the gallbladder and the inferior vena cava divides the liver into two lobes (Fig. 157, p. 115).

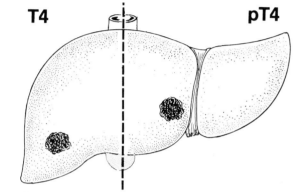

**Fig. 166**

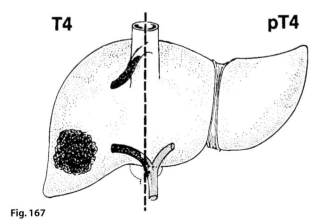

**Fig. 167**

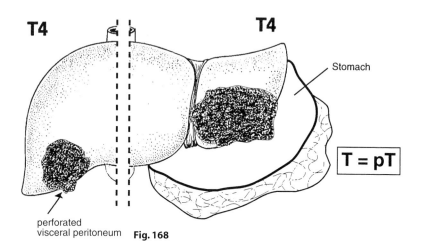

**T4**            **T4**

Stomach

T = pT

perforated
visceral peritoneum    **Fig. 168**

## N – Regional Lymph Nodes

NX    Regional lymph nodes cannot be assessed
N0    No regional lymph node metastasis
N1    Regional lymph node metastasis (Fig. 169)

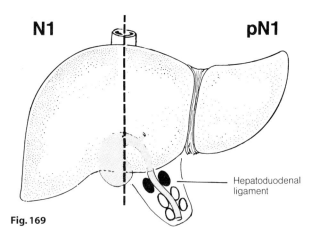

**N1**            **pN1**

Hepatoduodenal
ligament

**Fig. 169**

## pTN Pathological Classification

The pT and pN categories correspond to the T and N categories.

pN0   Histological examination of a regional lymphadenectomy specimen will ordinarily include 3 or more lymph nodes.

# Gallbladder (ICD-O C23.9)

## Rules for Classification

The classification applies only to carcinomas. There should be histological confirmation of the disease.

## Regional Lymph Nodes (Fig. 170)

The regional lymph nodes are the cystic duct node and the pericholedochal, hilar, peripancreatic (head only), periduodenal, periportal, coeliac and superior mesenteric nodes.

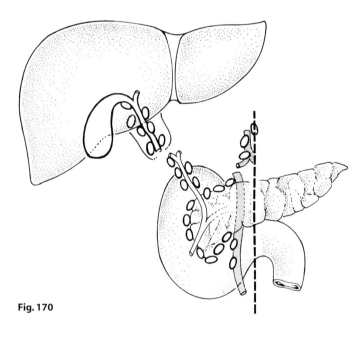

**Fig. 170**

## TN Clinical Classification

### T – Primary Tumour

TX    Primary tumour cannot be assessed
T0    No evidence of primary tumour
Tis   Carcinoma in situ

T1    Tumour invades lamina propria or muscle layer (Fig. 171)
      T1a   Tumour invades lamina propria
      T1b   Tumour invades muscle layer

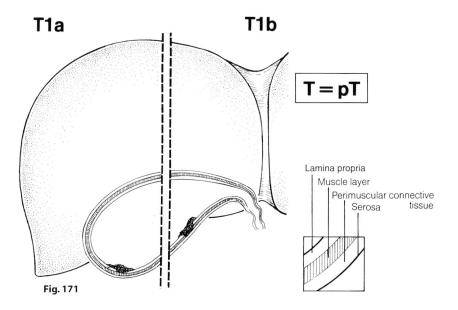

**T1a**

**T1b**

$T = pT$

Lamina propria
Muscle layer
Perimuscular connective tissue
Serosa

**Fig. 171**

T2    Tumour invades perimuscular connective tissue, no extension beyond serosa or into liver (Fig. 172)

T3    Tumour perforates serosa (visceral peritoneum) or directly invades into one adjacent organ or both (extension 2 cm or less into liver) (Fig. 173, 174)

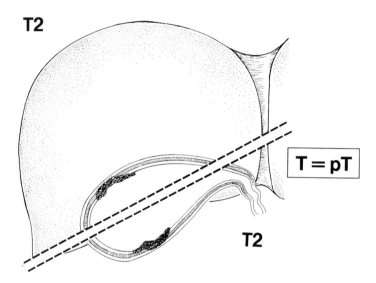

**Fig. 172**

**T3**

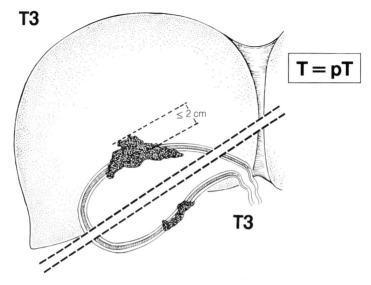

$$\boxed{T = pT}$$

≤ 2 cm

**T3**

Fig. 173

**T3**  **pT3**

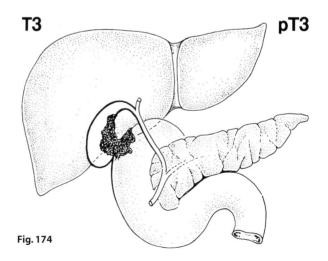

Fig. 174

T4    Tumour extends more than 2 cm into liver and/or into two or more adjacent organs (stomach, duodenum, colon, pancreas, omentum, extrahepatic bile ducts, any involvement of liver) (Figs. 175, 176)

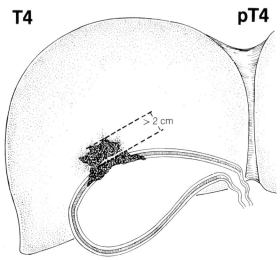

**Fig. 175**

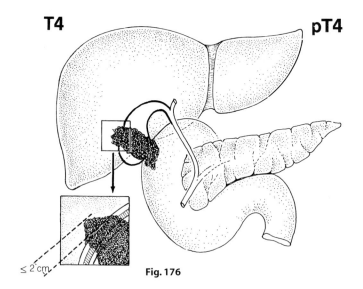

**Fig. 176**

## N – Regional Lymph Nodes

NX   Regional lymph nodes cannot be assessed
N0   No regional lymph node metastasis
N1   Metastasis in cystic duct, pericholedochal, and/or hilar lymph nodes (i.e. in the hepatoduodenal ligament) (Figs. 177, 178)

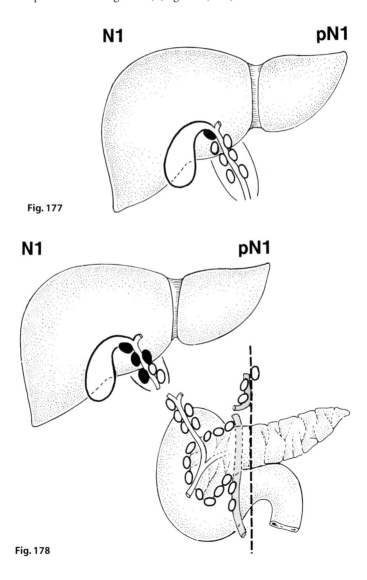

**Fig. 177**

**Fig. 178**

N2    Metastasis in peripancreatic (head only), periduodenal, periportal, coeliac and/or superior mesenteric lymph nodes (Fig. 179)

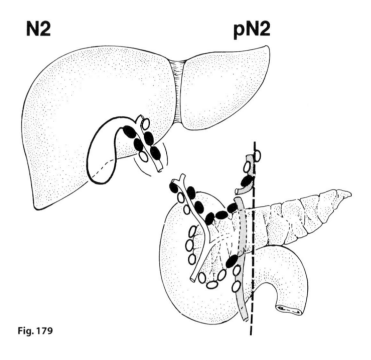

**N2**                    **pN2**

**Fig. 179**

## pTN Pathological Classification

The pT and pN categories correspond to the T and N categories.

pN0    Histological examination of a regional lymphadenectomy specimen will ordinarily include 3 or more lymph nodes.

# Extrahepatic Bile Ducts (ICD-O C24.0)

## Rules for Classification

The classification applies only to carcinomas of extrahepatic bile ducts and those of choledochal cysts. There should be histological confirmation of the disease.

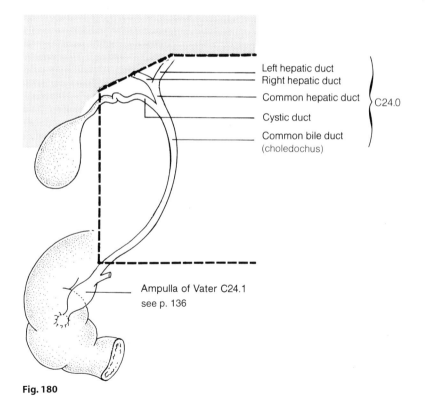

Left hepatic duct
Right hepatic duct
Common hepatic duct ⎫
Cystic duct          ⎬ C24.0
Common bile duct     ⎭
(choledochus)

Ampulla of Vater C24.1
see p. 136

**Fig. 180**

## Anatomical Subsites (Fig. 180)

1. Right hepatic duct
2. Left hepatic duct
3. Common hepatic duct
4. Cystic duct
5. Common bile duct (choledochus)

## Regional Lymph Nodes (see Fig. 170, p. 124)

The regional lymph nodes are the cystic duct, pericholedochal, hilar, peripancreatic (head only), periduodenal, periportal, coeliac and superior mesenteric nodes.

## TN Clinical Classification

### T – Primary Tumour

TX    Primary tumour cannot be assessed
T0    No evidence of primary tumour
Tis   Carcinoma in situ
T1    Tumour invades subepithelial connective tissue or fibromuscular layer
    T1a    Tumour invades subepithelial connective tissue (Fig. 181)
    T1b    Tumour invades fibromuscular layer (Fig. 181)
T2    Tumour invades perifibromuscular connective tissue (Fig. 182)

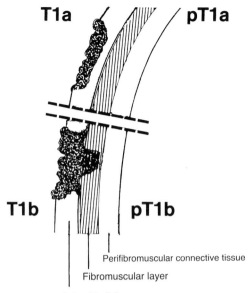

**T1a**      **pT1a**

**T1b**      **pT1b**

Perifibromuscular connective tissue

Fibromuscular layer

Subepithelial connective tissue

**Fig. 181**

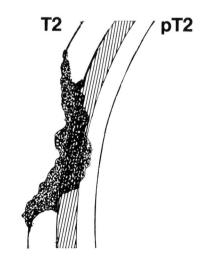

**T2**    **pT2**

**Fig. 182**

T3    Tumour invades adjacent structures: liver, pancreas, duodenum, gall-
       bladder, colon, stomach (Figs. 183, 184)

**T3**                          **pT3**

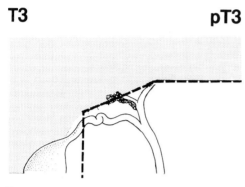

**Fig. 183**

**T3**                    **pT3**

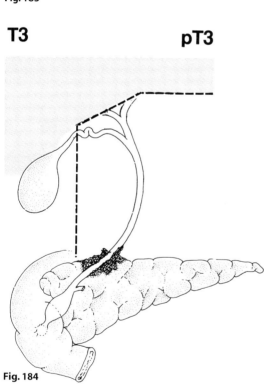

**Fig. 184**

## N – Regional Lymph Nodes

NX    Regional lymph nodes cannot be assessed

N0    No regional lymph node metastasis

N1    Metastasis in cystic duct, pericholedochal and/or hilar lymph nodes (i.e. in the hepatoduodenal ligament) (see Figs. 177, 178, p. 127)

N2    Metastasis in peripancreatic (head only), periduodenal, periportal, coeliac, superior mesenteric and/or posterior peripancreaticoduodenal lymph nodes (see Fig. 179, p. 128)

## pTN Pathological Classification

The pT and pN categories correspond to the T and N categories.

pN0    Histological examination of a regional lymphadenectomy specimen will ordinarily include 3 or more lymph nodes.

# Ampulla of Vater (ICD-O C24.1) (Fig. 185)

## Rules for Classification

The classification applies only to carcinomas. There should be histological confirmation of the disease.

## Regional Lymph Nodes (Fig. 186)

The regional lymph nodes are:
**Superior**    Superior to head (1) and body (2) of the pancreas
**Inferior**    Inferior to head (3) and body (4) of the pancreas

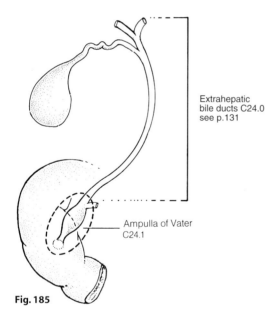

Extrahepatic
bile ducts C24.0
see p.131

Ampulla of Vater
C24.1

**Fig. 185**

**Anterior**     Anterior pancreaticoduodenal (5), pyloric (6, not shown in Fig. 186) and proximal mesenteric (7)

**Posterior**     Posterior pancreaticoduodenal (8), common bile duct (9) and proximal mesenteric (7)

**Note:**     The splenic lymph nodes and those at the tail of the pancreas are not regional; metastases to these lymph nodes are coded M1.

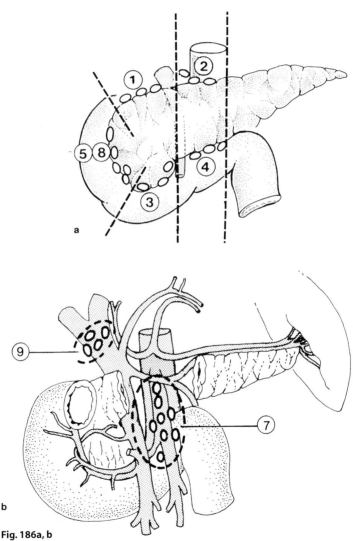

**Fig. 186a, b**

## TNM Clinical Classification

### T – Primary Tumour

TX    Primary tumour cannot be assessed
T0    No evidence of primary tumour
Tis   Carcinoma in situ

T1    Tumour limited to ampulla of Vater or sphincter of Oddi (Fig. 187)
T2    Tumour invades duodenal wall (Fig. 188)

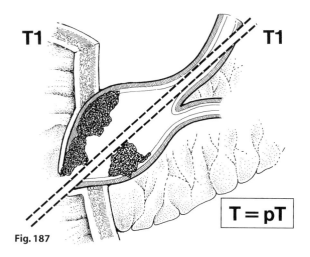

**Fig. 187**

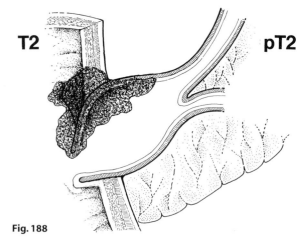

**Fig. 188**

T3    Tumour invades 2 cm or less into pancreas (Fig. 189)
T4    Tumour invades more than 2 cm into pancreas and/or into other adjacent organs (Fig. 190)

**T3**                                              **pT3**

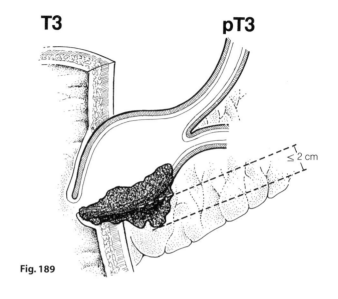

**Fig. 189**

**T4**                                              **pT4**

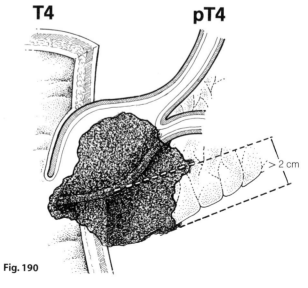

**Fig. 190**

## N – Regional Lymph Nodes

NX    Regional lymph nodes cannot be assessed
N0    No regional lymph node metastasis
N1    Regional lymph node metastasis (Figs. 191, 192)

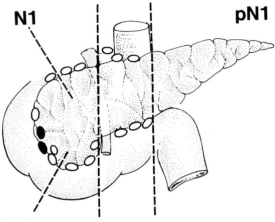

**Fig. 191**

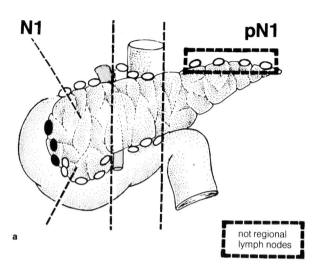

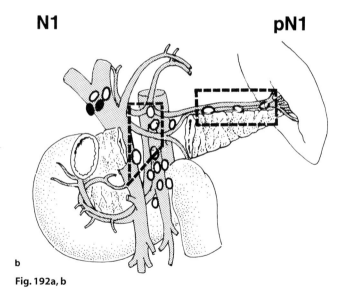

**Fig. 192a, b**

## M – Distant Metastasis

MX  Distant metastasis cannot be assessed
M0  No distant metastasis
M1  Distant metastasis (Fig. 193) (includes metastasis in splenic lymph nodes and/or those at the tail of the pancreas)

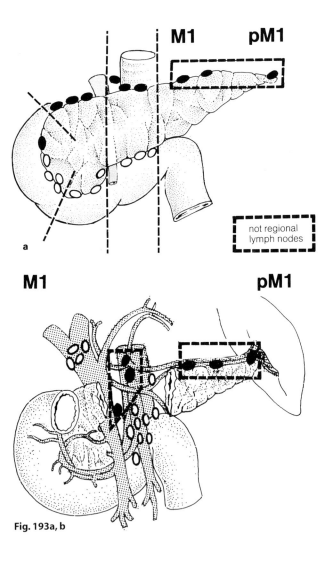

**Fig. 193a, b**

## pTNM Pathological Classification

The pT, pN and pM categories correspond to the T, N and M categories.

pN0    Histological examination of a regional lymphadenectomy specimen will ordinarily include 10 or more lymph nodes.

# Pancreas (ICD-0 C25.0-2,8)

## Rules for Classification

The classification applies only to carcinomas of the exocrine pancreas. There should be histological or cytological confirmation of the disease.

## Anatomical Subsites (Fig. 194)

1. Head of pancreas[1] (C25.0)
2. Body of pancreas[2] (C25.1)
3. Tail of pancreas[3] (C25.2)
4. Entire pancreas (C25.8)

**Notes:** 1. Tumours of the head of the pancreas are those arising to the right of the left border of the superior mesenteric vein. The uncinate process is considered as part of the head.
2. Tumours of the body are those arising between the left border of the superior mesenteric vein and the left border of the aorta.
3. Tumours of the tail are those arising between the left border of the aorta and the hilum of the spleen.

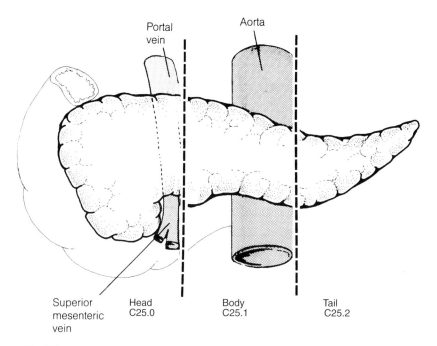

**Fig. 194**

## Regional Lymph Nodes (Fig. 195)

The regional lymph nodes are the peripancreatic nodes which may be subdivided as follows:

**Superior**     Superior to head (1) and body (2)

**Inferior**     Inferior to head (3) and body (4)

**Anterior**     Anterior pancreaticoduodenal (5), pyloric (for tumours of head only) (6, not shown in Fig. 195) and proximal mesenteric (7)

**Posterior**    Posterior pancreaticoduodenal (8), common bile duct (9) and proximal mesenteric (7)

**Splenic**      Hilum of spleen (10) and tail of pancreas (11) (for tumours of body and tail only)

**Celiac** (12)   (for tumours of head only)

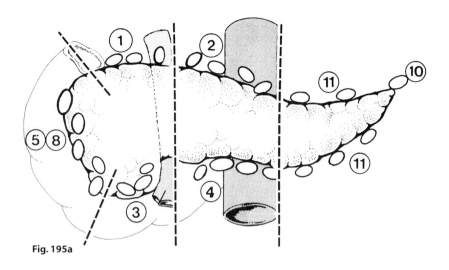

Fig. 195a

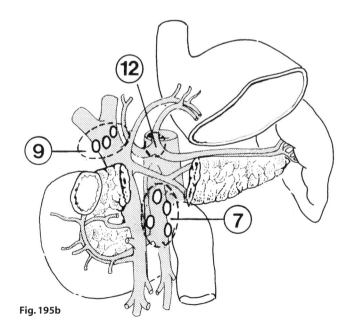

Fig. 195b

## TN Clinical Classification

### T – Primary Tumour

TX    Primary tumour cannot be assessed
T0    No evidence of primary tumour
Tis    Carcinoma in situ

T1    Tumour limited to the pancreas, 2 cm or less in greatest dimension
      (Fig. 196)

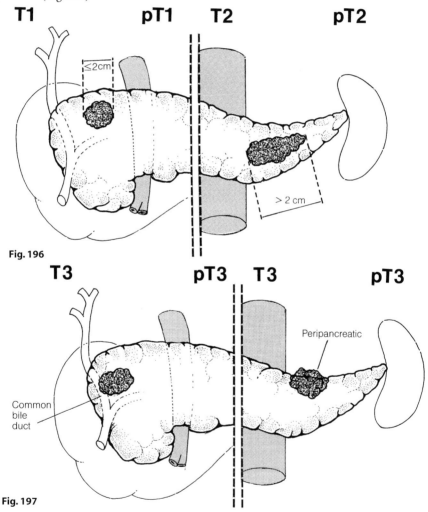

Fig. 196

Fig. 197

T2    Tumour limited to the pancreas, more than 2 cm in greatest dimension (Fig. 196)

T3    Tumour extends directly into any of the following: duodenum, bile duct, peripancreatic tissues[1] (Figs. 197, 198)

T4    Tumour extends directly into any of the following: stomach, spleen, colon, adjacent large vessels[2] (Fig. 199)

**Note:**    1. Peripancreatic tissues include the surrounding retroperitoneal fat (retroperitoneal soft tissue or retroperitoneal space), including mesentery (mesenteric fat), mesocolon, greater and lesser omentum, and peritoneum. Direct invasion to bile ducts and duodenum includes involvement of ampulla of Vater.

2. Adjacent large vessels are the portal vein, coeliac artery, and superior mesenteric and common hepatic arteries and veins (not splenic vessels).

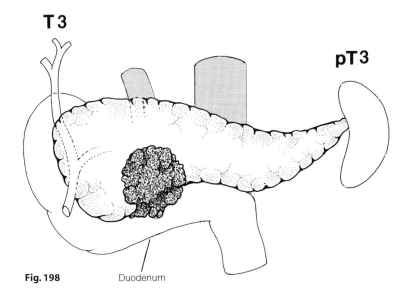

**T 3**

**pT 3**

**Fig. 198**          Duodenum

# T4

# pT4

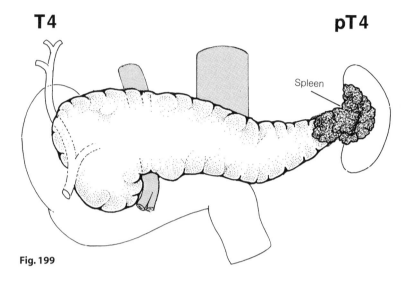

Spleen

**Fig. 199**

## N – Regional Lymph Nodes

NX    Regional lymph nodes cannot be assessed
N0    No regional lymph node metastasis
N1    Regional lymph node metastasis
    N1a    Metastasis in a single regional lymph node (Fig. 200)
    N1b    Metastasis in multiple regional lymph nodes (Fig. 201)

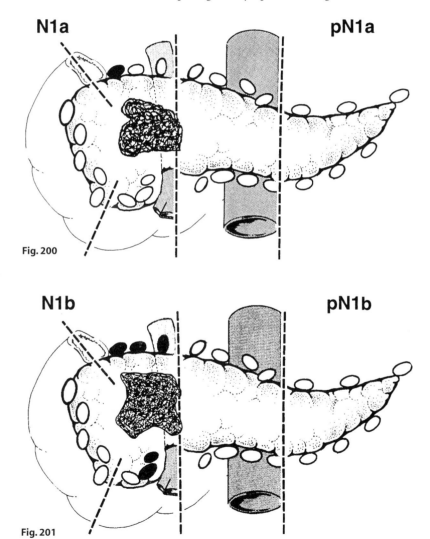

**N1a**　　　　　　　　　　　　　　　**pN1a**

Fig. 200

**N1b**　　　　　　　　　　　　　　　**pN1b**

Fig. 201

**N1b** 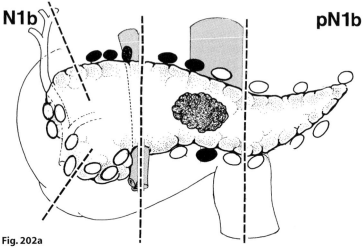 **pN1b**

Fig. 202a

**N1b** 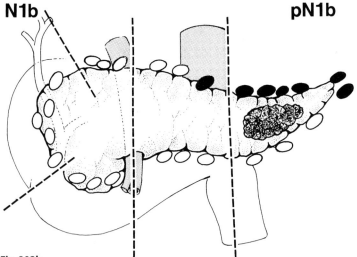 **pN1b**

Fig. 202b

## pTN Pathological Classification

The pT and pN categories correspond to the T and N categories.

pN0    Histological examination of a regional lymphadenectomy specimen will ordinarily include 10 or more lymph nodes.

# Lung and Pleural Tumours

## Introductory Notes

The classifications apply to carcinomas of the lung and malignant mesothelioma of the pleura.

## Regional Lymph Nodes (Figs. 203, 204)

The regional lymph nodes are the intrathoracic, scalene and supraclavicular nodes.
The intrathoracic nodes include:

a) *Mediastinal nodes* (Fig. 203b, c; black in Fig. 203a; Fig. 204):
- (1)   highest(superior) mediastinal
- (2)   paratracheal (upper paratracheal)
- (3)   pretracheal
- (3a)  anterior mediastinal
- (3p)  retrotracheal (posterior mediastinal)
- (4)   tracheobronchial (lower paratracheal) (including azygos nodes)
- (5)   subaortic (aortic window)
- (6)   para-aortic (ascending aorta or phrenic)
- (7)   subcarinal
- (8)   paraoesophageal (below carina)
- (9)   pulmonary ligament

b)   *Peribronchial and hilar nodes* (Fig. 203a: Fig. 204):
- (10)  hilar (main bronchus)
- (11)  interlobar
- (12)  lobar
- (13)  segmental
- (14)  subsegmental

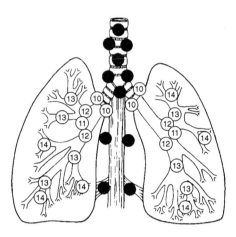

**Fig. 203a**

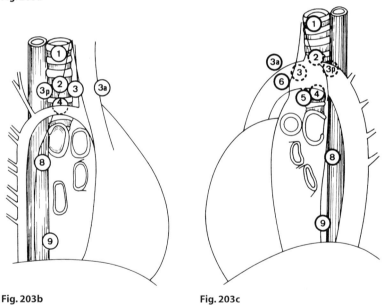

**Fig. 203b**                          **Fig. 203c**

**Fig. 203a–c.** Lymph node map of Naruke. [Modified from Naruke T, Suemasu K, Ishikawa S (1978) Lymph node mapping and curability at various levels of metastasis in resected lung cancer. J Thorac Cardiovasc Surg 76: 832-839]

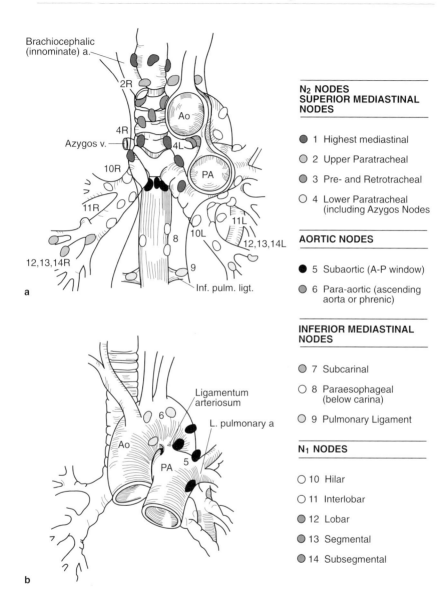

**Fig. 204a, b.**   Regional lymph nodes for lung cancer. Used with the permission of the American Joint Committee on Cancer (AJCC), Chicago, Illinois. The original source for the material is the AJCC Cancer Staging Manual, 5th edition (1997) published by Lippincott-Raven Publishers, Philadelphia, Pennsylvania.

# Lung Carcinomas (ICD-O C34)

## Rules for Classification

The classification applies only to carcinomas. There should be histological confirmation of the disease and division of cases by histological type.

## Anatomical Subsites (Fig. 205)

1. Main bronchus (C34.0)
2. Upper lobe (C34.1)
3. Middle lobe (C34.2)
4. Lower lobe (C34.3)

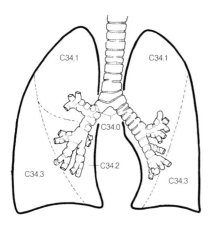

**Fig. 205**

# TNM Clinical Classification

## T – Primary Tumour

TX    Primary tumour cannot be assessed, *or* tumour proven by the presence of malignant cells in sputum or bronchial washings but not visualized by imaging or bronchoscopy

T0    No evidence of primary tumour

Tis    Carcinoma in situ

T1    Tumour 3 cm or less in greatest dimension, surrounded by lung or visceral pleura, without bronchoscopic evidence of invasion more proximal than the lobar bronchus (i.e. not in the main bronchus)[1] (Fig. 206)

T2    Tumour with *any* of the following features of size or extent (Fig. 207):
 –    More than 3 cm in greatest dimension
 –    Involves main bronchus, 2 cm or more distal to the carina
 –    Invades visceral pleura
 –    Associated with atelectasis or obstructive pneumonitis which extends to the hilar region but does not involve the entire lung

T3    Tumour of any size which directly invades any of the following: chest wall (including superior sulcus tumours), diaphragm, mediastinal pleura, parietal pericardium; *or* tumour in the main bronchus less than 2 cm distal to the carina[1] but without involvement of the carina; *or* associated atelectasis or obstructive pneumonitis of the entire lung (Fig. 208)

T4    Tumour of any size which invades any of the following: mediastinum, heart (Figs. 209, 210), great vessels (Figs. 209, 211, 212), trachea, oesophagus (Fig. 213), vertebral body (Fig. 214), carina; *or* separate tumour nodule(s) in the same lobe (Fig. 215); *or* tumour with malignant pleural effusion[2] (Figs. 216, 217).

**Notes:**    1. The uncommon superficial spreading tumour of any size with its invasive component limited to the bronchial wall, which may extend proximal to the main bronchus, is also classified as T1.

2. Most pleural effusions associated with lung cancer are due to tumour. In a few patients, however, multiple cytopathological examinations of pleural fluid are negative for tumour, and the fluid is non-bloody and is not an exudate. Where these elements and clinical judgement dictate that the effusion is not related to the tumour, the effusion should be excluded as a staging element and the patient should be classified as T1, T2 or T3.

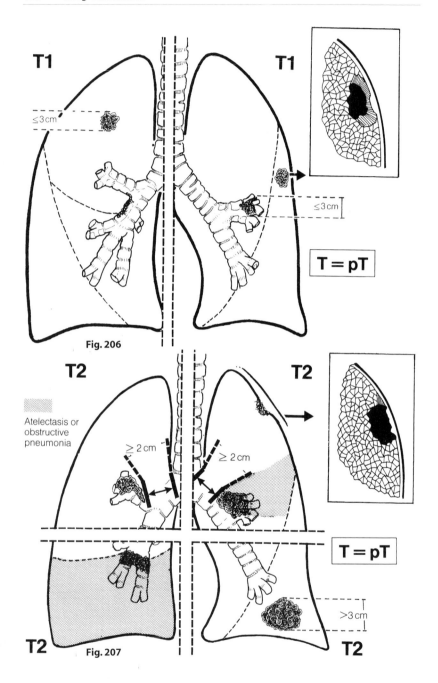

**T1**

≤3cm

**T1**

≤3cm

T = pT

**Fig. 206**

**T2**

Atelectasis or obstructive pneumonia

**T2**

≥ 2 cm

≥ 2 cm

T = pT

>3cm

**T2**

**T2**

**Fig. 207**

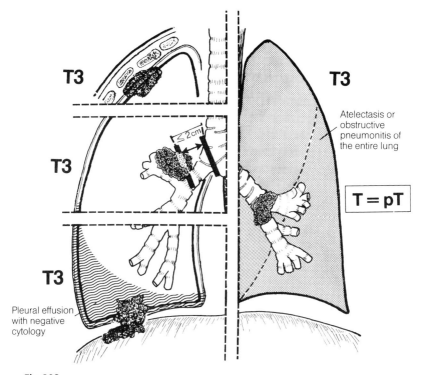

**T3**

**T3**

**T3**

**T3**

Atelectasis or
obstructive
pneumonitis of
the entire lung

$T = pT$

Pleural effusion
with negative
cytology

**Fig. 208**

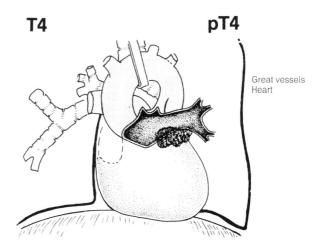

**T4**

**pT4**

Great vessels
Heart

**Fig. 209**

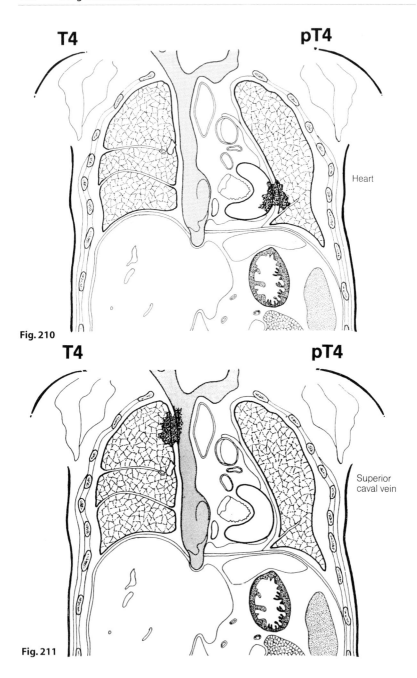

**T4**                                    **pT4**

Heart

**Fig. 210**

**T4**                                    **pT4**

Superior
caval vein

**Fig. 211**

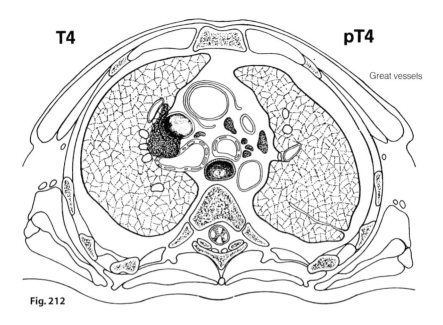

**T4**    **pT4**

Great vessels

**Fig. 212**

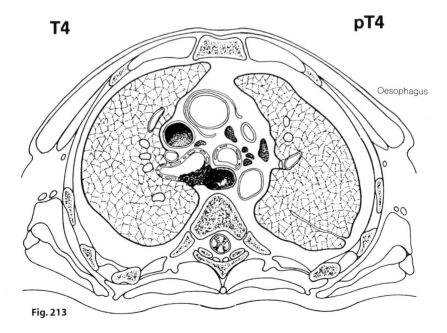

**T4**    **pT4**

Oesophagus

**Fig. 213**

**T4**                                              **pT4**

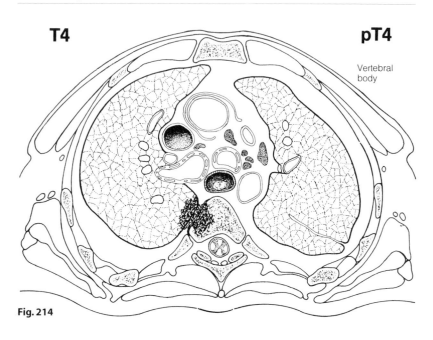

Vertebral
body

**Fig. 214**

**T4**                                              **M1**

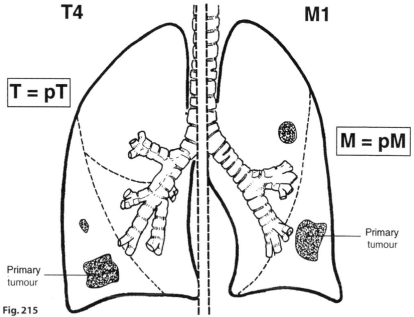

T = pT

M = pM

Primary
tumour

Primary
tumour

**Fig. 215**

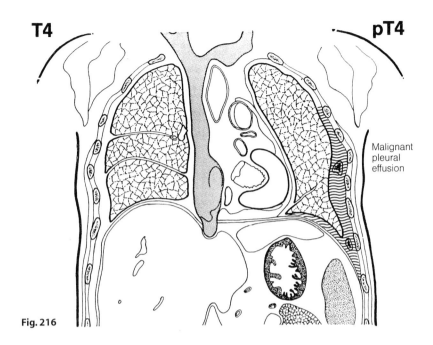

**T4**

**pT4**

Malignant
pleural
effusion

**Fig. 216**

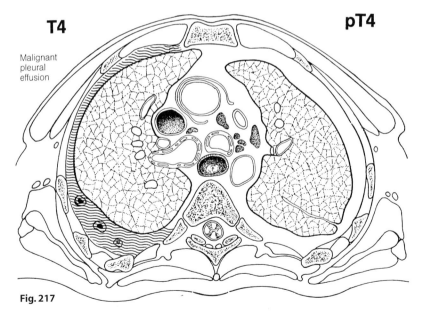

**T4**

**pT4**

Malignant
pleural
effusion

**Fig. 217**

## N – Regional Lymph Nodes

NX    Regional lymph nodes cannot be assessed

N0    No regional lymph node metastasis

N1    Metastasis in ipsilateral peribronchial and/or ipsilateral hilar lymph nodes and/or intrapulmonary nodes including involvement by direct extension (Fig. 218)

N2    Metastasis in ipsilateral mediastinal and/or subcarinal lymph node(s) (Fig. 219)

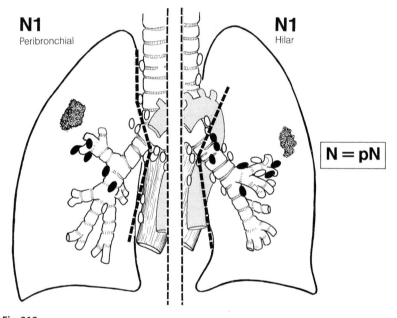

**N1**
Peribronchial

**N1**
Hilar

N = pN

**Fig. 218**

**N2**

**N2**

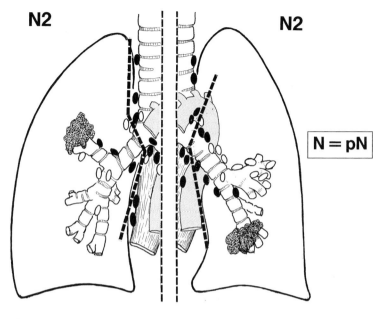

N = pN

Fig. 219

N3    Metastasis in contralateral mediastinal, contralateral hilar, ipsilateral or contralateral scalene or supraclavicular lymph node(s) (Fig. 220)

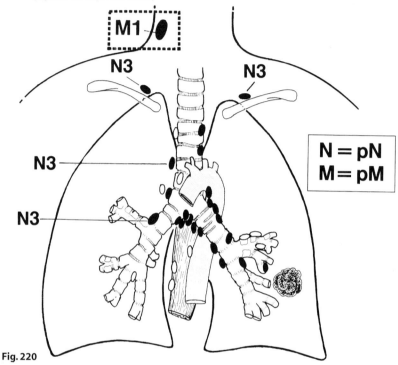

**Fig. 220**

## M – Distant Metastasis

MX    Distant metastasis cannot be assessed

M0    No distant metastasis

M1    Distant metastasis, includes separate tumour nodule(s) in a different lobe (ipsilateral or contralateral) (see Fig. 215, p. 162)

## pTNM Pathological Classification

The pT, pN and pM categories correspond to the T, N and M categories.

pN0    Histological examination of hilar and mediastinal lymphadenectomy specimen(s) will ordinarily include 6 or more lymph nodes.

# Pleural Mesothelioma (ICD-O C38.4)

## Rules for Classification

The classification applies only to malignant mesothelioma of the pleura. There should be histological confirmation of the disease.

## TNM Clinical Classification

### T – Primary Tumour

TX    Primary tumour cannot be assessed
T0    No evidence of primary tumour

T1    Tumour limited to ipsilateral parietal and/or visceral pleura
      (Fig. 221, 222)

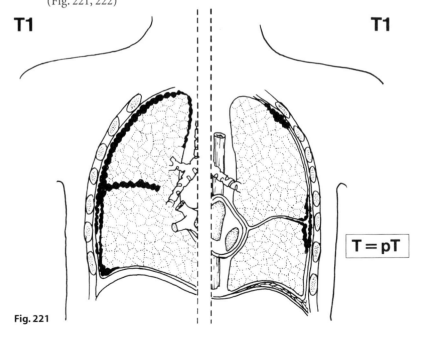

**T1**                                                        **T1**

T = pT

**Fig. 221**

T2    Tumour invades any of the following: ipsilateral lung, endothoracic fascia, diaphragm, pericardium (Fig. 223, 224)

T3    Tumour invades any of the following: ipsilateral chest wall muscle, ribs, mediastinal organs or tissues (Fig. 225)

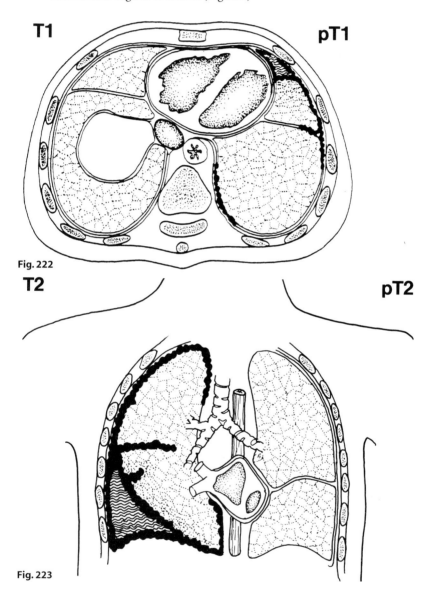

**T1**    **pT1**

**Fig. 222**

**T2**    **pT2**

**Fig. 223**

**T2**
**pT2**

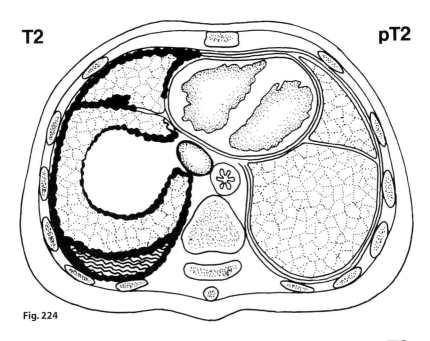

Fig. 224

**T3**
**pT3**

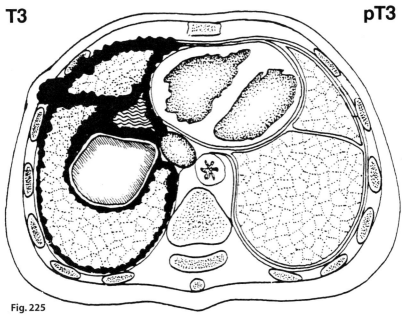

Fig. 225

T4      Tumour directly extends to any of the following: contralateral pleura, contralateral lung, peritoneum, intra-abdominal organs, cervical tissues (Figs. 226, 227)

**T4**                          **pT4**

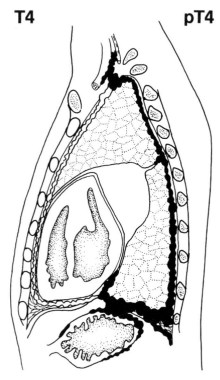

**Fig. 226**

**T4**  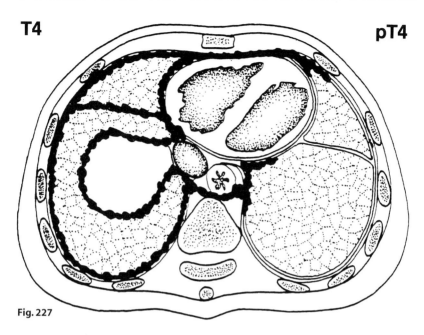  **pT4**

**Fig. 227**

## N – Regional Lymph Nodes

NX   Regional lymph nodes cannot be assessed

N0   No regional lymph node metastasis

N1   Metastasis in ipsilateral peribronchial and/or ipsilateral hilar lymph nodes, including involvement by direct extension (see Fig. 218, p. 164)

N2   Metastasis in ipsilateral mediastinal and/or subcarinal lymph node(s) (see Fig. 219, p. 165)

N3   Metastasis in contralateral mediastinal, contralateral hilar, ipsilateral or contralateral scalene, or supraclavicular lymph node(s) (see Fig. 220, p 166)

## M – Distant Metastasis

See p. 166 (Fig. 220) and Fig. 215 (p. 162).

## pTNM Pathological Classification

The pT, pN and pM categories correspond to the T, N and M categories.

Six lymph nodes ordinarily are included in a hilar or mediastinal lymphadenectomy specimen. The designation pN0 is usually based on this figure.

# Tumours of Bone and Soft Tissues

## Introductory Notes

The following sites are included:
    Bone
    Soft tissues

## Regional Lymph Nodes

The regional lymph nodes are those appropriate to the site of the primary tumour (see Fig. 479, p. 371). The definitions of the N categories for all tumours of bone and soft tissues are:

### N – Regional Lymph Nodes

NX    Regional lymph nodes cannot be assessed
N0    No regional lymph node metastasis
N1    Regional lymph node metastasis

# Bone (ICD-O C40, C41)

## Rules for Classification

The classification applies to all primary malignant bone tumours except malignant lymphomas, multiple myeloma, surface/juxtacortical osteosarcoma and juxtacortical chondrosarcoma. There should be histological confirmation of the disease and division of cases by histological type and grade.

## T Clinical Classification

### T – Primary Tumour

TX     Primary tumour cannot be assessed
T0     No evidence of primary tumour

T1     Tumour confined within the cortex (Fig. 228)
T2     Tumour invades beyond the cortex (Fig. 229)

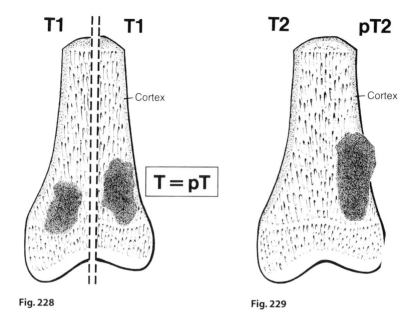

**Fig. 228**                **Fig. 229**

## pT Pathological Classification

The pT categories correspond to the T categories.

# Soft Tissues (ICD-O C38.1,2, C47-C49)

## Rules for Classification

There should be histological confirmation of the disease and division of cases by histological type and grade.

## Anatomical Sites

1. Connective, subcutaneous and other soft tissues, peripheral nerves (C47, C49)
2. Retroperitoneum (C48)
3. Mediastinum (C38.1,2)

## Histological Types of Tumour

The following histological types of malignant tumour are included, the appropriate ICD-O morphology rubrics being indicated:

| | |
|---|---|
| Alveolar soft-part sarcoma | 9581/3 |
| Angiosarcoma | 9120/3 |
| Epithelioid sarcoma | 8804/3 |
| Extraskeletal chondrosarcoma | 9220/3 |
| Extraskeletal osteosarcoma | 9180/3 |
| Fibrosarcoma | 8810/3 |
| Leiomyosarcoma | 8890/3 |
| Liposarcoma | 8850/3 |
| Malignant fibrous histiocytoma | 8830/3 |
| Malignant haemangiopericytoma | 9150/3 |
| Malignant mesenchymoma | 8990/3 |
| Malignant schwannoma | 9560/3 |
| Rhabdomyosarcoma | 8900/3 |
| Synovial sarcoma | 9040/3 |
| Sarcoma NOS (not otherwise specified) | 8800/3 |

The following histological types of tumour are not included: Kaposi sarcoma, dermatofibrosarcoma (protuberans), fibrosarcoma grade I (desmoid tumour) and sarcoma arising from the dura mater, brain, parenchymatous organs or hollow viscera.

## T Clinical Classification

### T – Primary Tumour

TX    Primary tumour cannot be assessed
T0    No evidence of primary tumour

T1    Tumour 5 cm or less in greatest dimension
       T1a   Superficial tumours[1] (Fig. 230)
       T1b   Deep tumours[1] (Fig. 231)
T2    Tumour more than 5 cm in greatest dimension
       T2a   Superficial tumour[1] (Fig. 230)
       T2b   Deep tumour[1] (Fig. 232)

**Note:**   1. Superficial tumour is located exclusively above the superficial fascia without invasion of the fascia; deep tumour is located either exclusively beneath the superficial fascia or superficial to the fascia with invasion of or through the fascia. Retroperitoneal, mediastinal and pelvic sarcomas are classified as deep tumours.

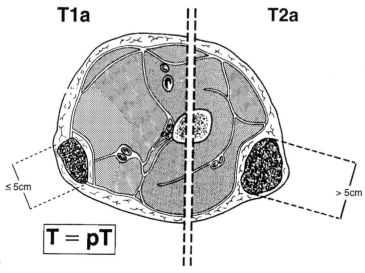

**T1a**          **T2a**

≤ 5cm           > 5cm

$$T = pT$$

**Fig. 230**

# T1b          pT1b

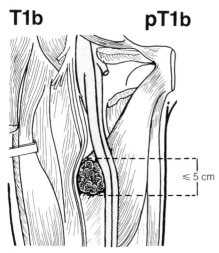

$\leqslant 5$ cm

**Fig. 231**

# T2b          pT2b

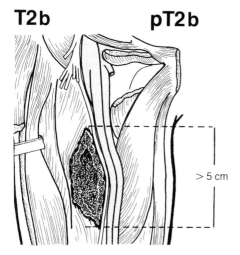

$> 5$ cm

**Fig. 232**

## pT Pathological Classification

The pT categories correspond to the T categories.

# Skin Tumours

## Introductory Notes

The classification applies to carcinomas of the skin excluding eyelid (see p. 329), vulva (see p. 214), penis (see p. 264) and to malignant melanoma of the skin including eyelid.

## Anatomical Sites

The following sites are identified by ICD-O topography rubrics:
1. Lip (excluding vermilion surface) (C44.0)
2. External ear (C44.2)
3. Other and unspecified parts of face (C44.3)
4. Scalp and neck (C44.4)
5. Trunk including anal margin and perianal skin (C44.5)
6. Upper limb and shoulder (C44.6)
7. Lower limb and hip (C44.7)
8. Scrotum (C63.2)

## Regional Lymph Nodes (Figs. 233, 234)

The regional lymph nodes are those appropriate to the site of the primary tumour.

### Unilateral Tumours

| | |
|---|---|
| Head, neck | Ipsilateral preauricular, submandibular, cervical and supraclavicular lymph nodes |
| Thorax | Ipsilateral axillary lymph nodes |
| Upper limb | Ipsilateral epitrochlear and axillary lymph nodes |
| Abdomen, loins and buttocks | Ipsilateral inguinal lymph nodes Lower limb |
| Lower Limb | Ipsilateral popliteal and inguinal lymph nodes |
| Anal margin and perianal skin | Ipsilateral inguinal lymph nodes |

C77.0

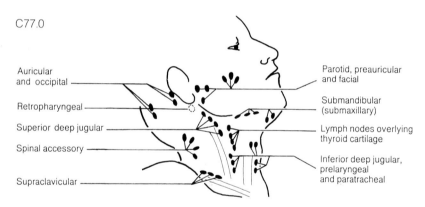

Auricular and occipital

Retropharyngeal

Superior deep jugular

Spinal accessory

Supraclavicular

Parotid, preauricular and facial

Submandibular (submaxillary)

Lymph nodes overlying thyroid cartilage

Inferior deep jugular, prelaryngeal and paratracheal

**Fig. 233**

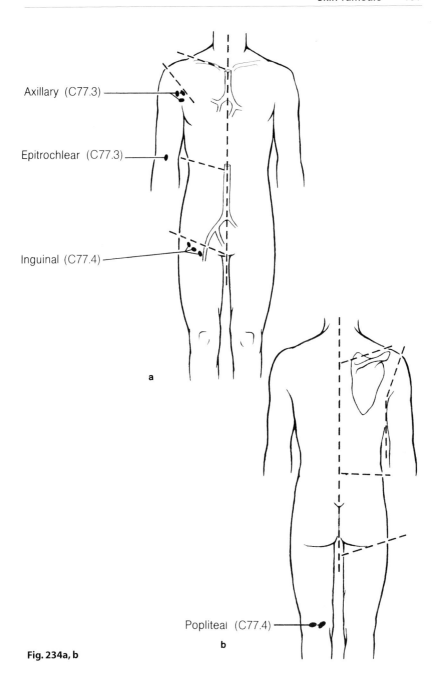

Axillary  (C77.3)

Epitrochlear  (C77.3)

Inguinal  (C77.4)

a

Popliteal  (C77.4)

b

Fig. 234a, b

*Tumours in the Boundary Zones Between the Above*

The lymph nodes pertaining to the regions on both sides of the boundary zone are considered to be regional lymph nodes. The following 4-cm-wide bands are considered as boundary zones (shown as interrupted lines in Figs. 234–239):

| *Between* | *Along* |
|---|---|
| Right/left | Midline |
| Head and neck/thorax | Clavicula-acromion-upper shoulder blade edge |
| Thorax/upper limb | Shoulder-axilla-shoulder |
| Thorax/abdomen, loins and buttocks | *Front:* middle between navel and costal arch |
| | *Back:* lower border of thoracic vertebrae (midtransverse axis) |
| Abdomen, loins and buttock/lower limb | Groin-trochanter-gluteal sulcus |

Any metastasis to other than the listed regional lymph nodes is considered as M1 (Figs. 235–238).

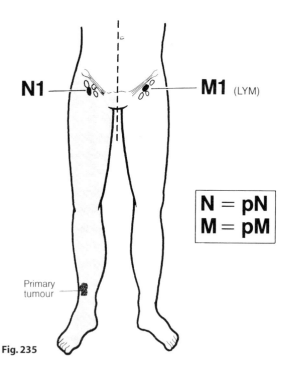

**Fig. 235**

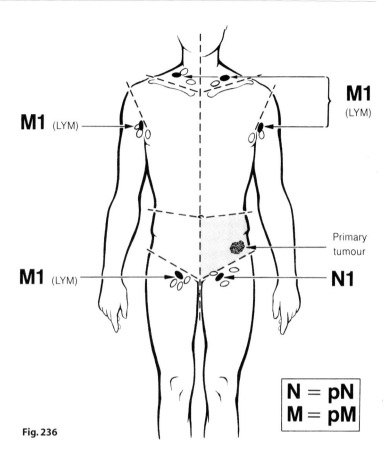

**M1** (LYM)

**M1** (LYM)

**M1** (LYM)

**M1** (LYM)

Primary tumour

**N1**

N = pN
M = pM

**Fig. 236**

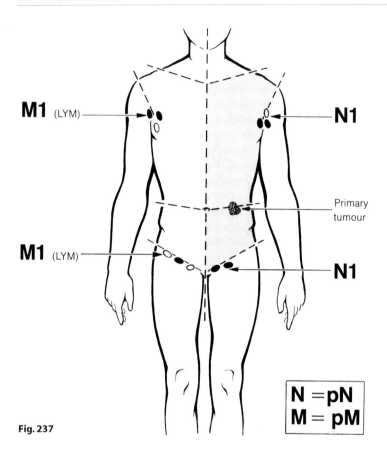

**M1** (LYM)

**M1** (LYM)

**N1**

Primary
tumour

**N1**

$$N = pN$$
$$M = pM$$

Fig. 237

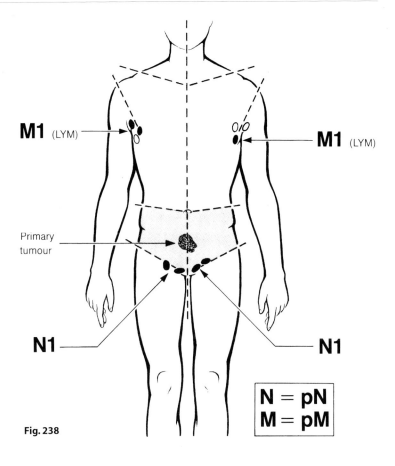

**M1** (LYM)

**M1** (LYM)

Primary
tumour

**N1**

**N1**

$$N = pN$$
$$M = pM$$

**Fig. 238**

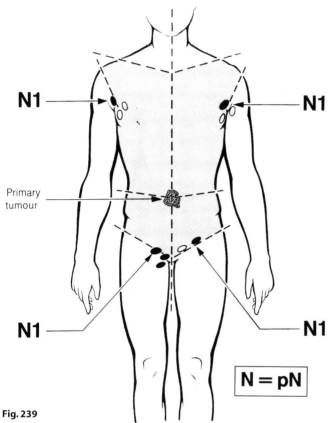

N1

N1

Primary
tumour

N1

N1

N = pN

**Fig. 239**

# Carcinoma of Skin (excluding eyelid, vulva and penis)
(ICD-O C44.0,2-9, C63.2)

## Rules for Classification

The classification applies only to carcinomas. There should be histological confirmation of the disease and division of cases by histological type.

## Regional Lymph Nodes

See p. 180.

## TNM Clinical Classification

### T – Primary Tumour

TX   Primary tumour cannot be assessed
T0   No evidence of primary tumour
Tis  Carcinoma in situ (Fig. 240)

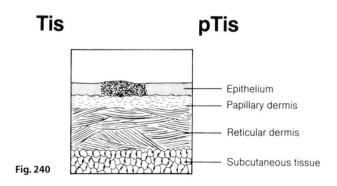

**Fig. 240**

T1    Tumour 2 cm or less in greatest dimension (Fig. 241)
T2    Tumour more than 2 cm but not more than 5 cm in greatest dimension
(Fig. 242)
T3    Tumour more than 5 cm in greatest dimension (Fig. 243)

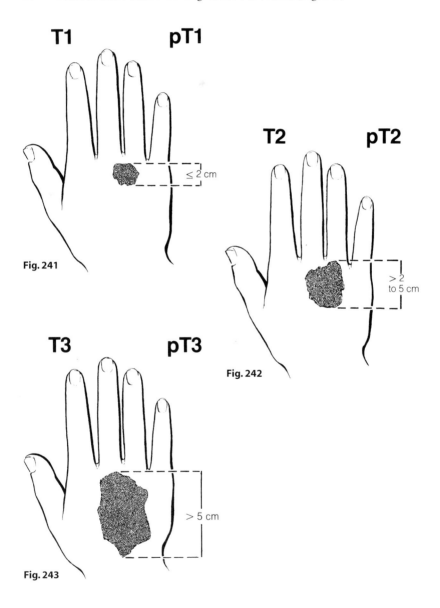

**T1**        **pT1**

≤ 2 cm

**Fig. 241**

**T2**        **pT2**

> 2
to 5 cm

**Fig. 242**

**T3**        **pT3**

> 5 cm

**Fig. 243**

T4    Tumour invades deep extradermal structures, i.e. cartilage, skeletal muscle or bone (Fig. 244)

**Note:**    In the case of multiple simultaneous tumours, the tumour with the highest T category is classified and the number of separate tumours is indicated in parenthesis, e.g. T2 (5) (Fig. 245)

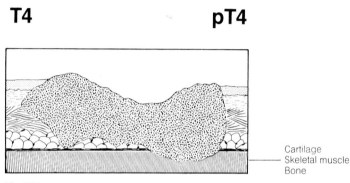

**Fig. 244**

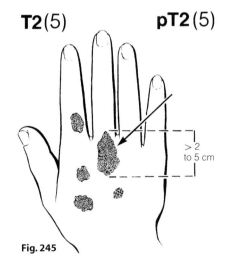

**Fig. 245**

## N – Regional Lymph Nodes

NX    Regional lymph nodes cannot be assessed
N0    No regional lymph node metastasis
N1    Regional lymph node metastasis (see Figs. 235–239, pp. 182–186)

## M – Distant Metastasis

MX    Distant metastasis cannot be assessed
M0    No distant metastasis
M1    Distant metastasis (see Figs. 235–238, pp. 182–185)

# pTNM Pathological Classification

The pT, pN and pM categories correspond to the T, N and M categories.

pN0    Histological examination of a regional lymphadenectomy specimen will
       ordinarily include 6 or more lymph nodes.

# Malignant Melanoma of Skin (ICD-O C44, C51.0, C60.9, C63.2)

## Rules for Classification

There should be histological confirmation of the disease.

## Regional Lymph Nodes

See p. 180.

## TNM Clinical Classification

### T – Primary Tumour

The extent of tumour is classified after excision, see pT, pp. 195–200

### N – Regional Lymph Nodes (See also Figs. 235–239, pp. 182–186)

- NX    Regional lymph nodes cannot be assessed
- N0    No regional lymph node metastasis
- N1    Metastasis 3 cm or less in greatest dimension in any regional lymph node(s) (Figs. 246, 247)
- N2    Metastasis more than 3 cm in greatest dimension in any regional lymph node(s) and/or in-transit metastasis
    - N2a    Metastasis more than 3 cm in greatest dimension in any regional lymph node(s) (Fig. 248)
    - N2b    In-transit metastasis (Figs. 249, 250)
    - N2c    Both (Fig. 251)

**Note:**    In-transit metastasis involves skin or subcutaneous tissue more than 2 cm from the primary tumour but not beyond the regional lymph nodes (see also Fig. 255, p. 197).

**N1**    **pN1**

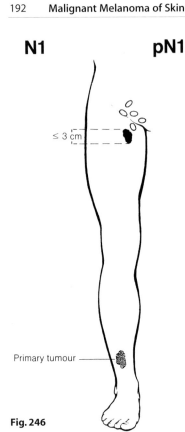

≤ 3 cm

Primary tumour ——

**Fig. 246**

**N1**    **pN1**

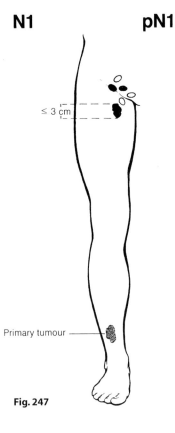

≤ 3 cm

Primary tumour ——

**Fig. 247**

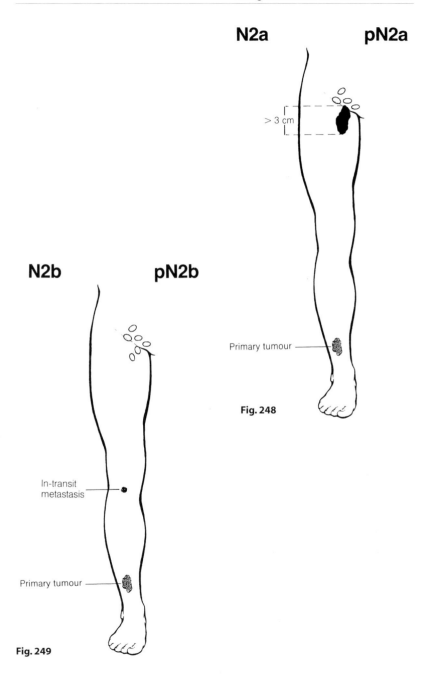

**N2a**                    **pN2a**

> 3 cm

Primary tumour

**Fig. 248**

**N2b**            **pN2b**

In-transit
metastasis

Primary tumour

**Fig. 249**

# N2b    pN2b

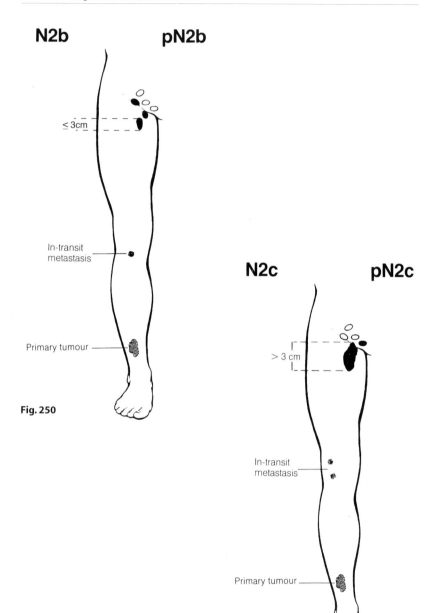

≤ 3cm

In-transit
metastasis

Primary tumour

**Fig. 250**

# N2c    pN2c

> 3 cm

In-transit
metastasis

Primary tumour

**Fig. 251**

## M – Distant Metastasis

MX    Distant metastasis cannot be assessed
M0    No distant metastasis
M1    Distant metastasis
       M1a Metastasis in skin or subcutaneous tissue or lymph node(s) beyond the regional lymph nodes (see Figs. 235–238, pp. 182–185)
       M1b Visceral metastasis

# pTNM Pathological Classification

## Introductory Note

The pT classification of malignant melanoma considers three histological criteria:
1. Tumour thickness (Breslow) according to the largest vertical diameter of the tumour in millimetres (Fig. 252) (melanoma cells within the epithelium of structures such as hair and sebaceous glands of the skin are not taken into consideration)
2. Clark "levels" (Fig. 253)
3. Absence or presence of satellites within 2 cm of the primary tumour (Fig. 254)

The definitive pT category is based on these three criteria (Fig. 256).
*In case of discrepancy* between tumour thickness and level, the pT category is based on the *less favourable finding.*

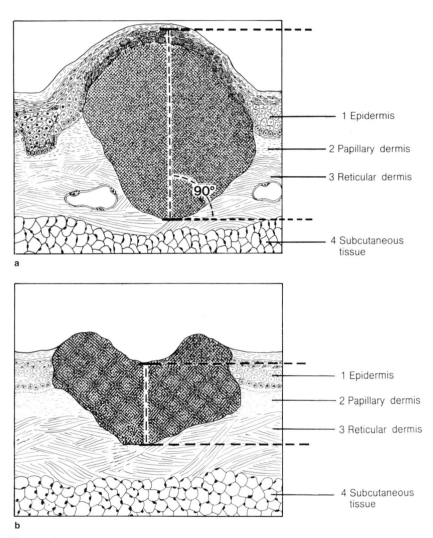

1 Epidermis

2 Papillary dermis

3 Reticular dermis

4 Subcutaneous tissue

a

1 Epidermis

2 Papillary dermis

3 Reticular dermis

4 Subcutaneous tissue

b

**Fig. 252a, b**

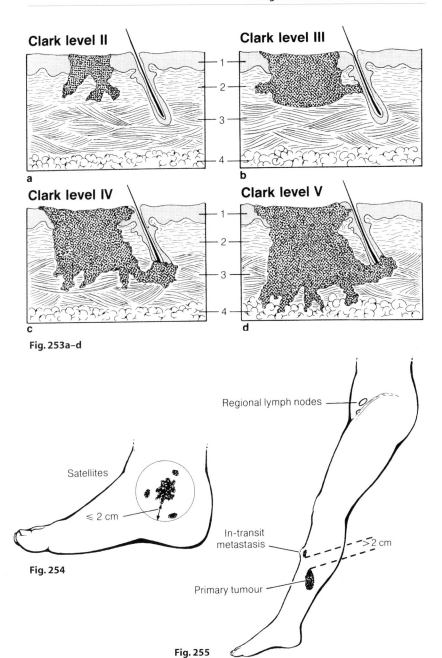

**Clark level II**

1
2
3
4

a

**Clark level III**

1
2
3
4

b

**Clark level IV**

1
2
3
4

c

**Clark level V**

1
2
3
4

d

Fig. 253a–d

Satellites

≤ 2 cm

Fig. 254

Regional lymph nodes

In-transit metastasis

> 2 cm

Primary tumour

Fig. 255

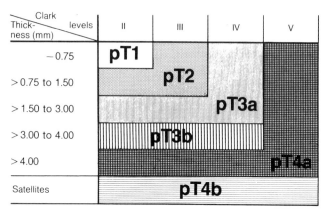

**Fig. 256**

## pT – Primary Tumour

pTX    Primary tumour cannot be assessed

pT0    No evidence of primary tumour

pTis   Melanoma in situ (Clark level I) (atypical melanocytic hyperplasia, severe mela-
       nocytic dysplasia, not an invasive malignant lesion)

pT1    Tumour 0.75 mm or less in thickness (Fig. 257) and invades the papillary
       dermis (Clark level II) (Fig. 253a)

pT2    Tumour more than 0.75 mm but not more than 1.5 mm in thickness (Fig.
       258) and/or invades the papillary-reticular dermal interface (Clark level
       III) (Fig. 253b)

pT3    Tumour more than 1.5 mm but not more than 4.0 mm in thickness (Figs.
       259, 260) and/or invades the reticular dermis (Clark level IV) (Fig. 253c)

    pT3a   Tumour more than 1.5 mm but not more than 3.0 mm in thick-
       ness (Fig. 259)

    pT3b   Tumour more than 3.0 mm but not more than 4.0 mm in thick-
       ness (Fig. 260)

# pT1

# pT2

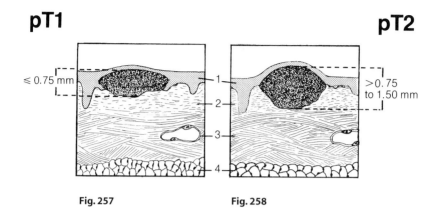

≤ 0.75 mm

>0.75 to 1.50 mm

**Fig. 257**          **Fig. 258**

# pT3a

# pT3b

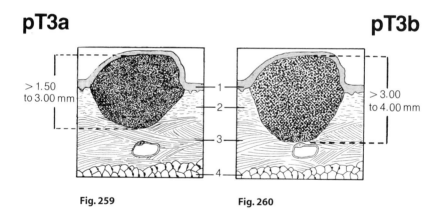

> 1.50 to 3.00 mm

> 3.00 to 4.00 mm

**Fig. 259**          **Fig. 260**

# pT4

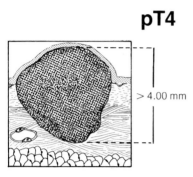

> 4.00 mm

**Fig. 261**

pT4    Tumour more than 4.0 mm in thickness (Fig. 261) and/or invades sub-
       cutaneous tissue (Clark level V) (Fig. 253d) and/or satellite(s) within
       2 cm of the primary tumour (Fig. 254)
       pT4a  Tumour more than 4.0 mm in thickness (Fig. 261) and/or invades
             subcutaneous tissue (Fig. 253d)
       pT4b  Satellite(s) within 2 cm of the primary tumour (Fig. 254)

**Note:**    In case of discrepancy between tumour thickness and level, the pT category is
         based on the less favourable finding (Fig. 256).

## pN – Regional Lymph Nodes

The pN categories correspond to the N categories.

pN0    Histological examination of a regional lymphadenectomy specimen will
       ordinarily include 6 or more lymph nodes.

## pM – Distant Metastasis

The pM categories correspond to the M categories.

# Breast Tumours (ICD-O C50)

## Rules for Classification

The classification applies only to carcinomas. There should be histological confirmation of the disease. The anatomical subsite of origin should be recorded but is not considered in classification.

In the case of multiple simultaneous tumours in one breast, the tumour with the highest T category should be used for classification. Simultaneous *bilateral* breast cancers should be classified independently to permit division of cases by histological type.

## Anatomical Sites and Subsites (Fig. 262)

1. Nipple (C50.0)
2. Central portion (C50.1)
3. Upper-inner quadrant (C50.2)
4. Lower-inner quadrant (C50.3)
5. Upper-outer quadrant (C50.4)
6. Lower-outer quadrant (C50.5)
7. Axillary tail (C50.6)

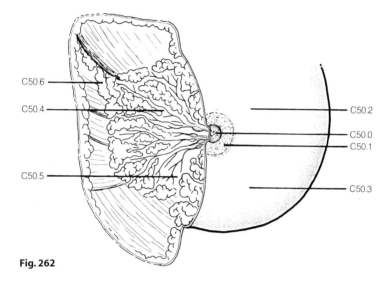

**Fig. 262**

## Regional Lymph Nodes (Fig. 263)

The regional lymph nodes are:
1. *Axillary* (ipsilateral): interpectoral (Rotter) nodes and lymph nodes along the axillary vein and its tributaries which may be divided into the following levels:
    i)   *Level I* (low-axilla): lymph nodes lateral to the lateral border of pectoralis minor muscle
    ii)  *Level II* (mid-axilla): lymph nodes between the medial and lateral borders of the pectoralis minor muscle and the interpectoral (Rotter) lymph nodes
    iii) *Level III* (apical axilla): lymph nodes medial to the medial margin of the pectoralis minor muscle including those designated as subclavicular, infraclavicular or apical

**Note:** Intramammary lymph nodes are coded as axillary lymph nodes.

2. *Internal mammary* (ipsilateral): lymph nodes in the intercostal spaces along the edge of the sternum in the endothoracic fascia.

Any other lymph node metastasis is coded as a distant metastasis (M1), including supraclavicular, cervical or contralateral internal mammary lymph nodes (see Fig. 275, p. 210).

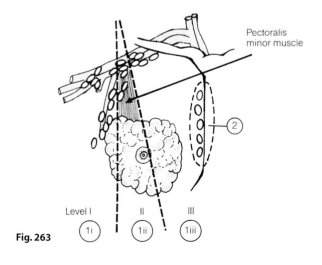

Pectoralis
minor muscle

Level I     II     III

**Fig. 263**     1i     1ii     1iii     2

# TN Clinical Classification

## T – Primary Tumour

TX    Primary tumour cannot be assessed
T0    No evidence of primary tumour
Tis   Carcinoma in situ: intraductal carcinoma, or lobular carcinoma in situ, or Paget disease of the nipple with no tumour (Fig. 264)

> **Note:**    Paget disease associated with a tumour is classified according to the size of the tumour.

T1    Tumour 2 cm or less in greatest dimension (Fig. 266)
      T1mic   Microinvasion 0.1 cm or less in greatest dimension (Fig. 265)

> **Note:**    Microinvasion is the extension of cancer cells beyond the basement membrane into the adjacent tissues with no focus more than 0.1 cm in greatest dimension. When there are multiple foci of microinvasion, the size of only the largest focus is used to classify the microinvasion. (Do not use the sum of all the individual foci.) The presence of multiple foci of microinvasion should be noted, as it is with multiple larger invasive carcinomas.

      T1a    More than 0.1 cm but not more than 0.5 cm in greatest dimension (Fig. 266)
      T1b    More than 0.5 cm but not more than 2 cm in greatest dimension (Fig. 266)
      T1c    More than 1 cm but not more than 2 cm in greatest dimension (Fig. 266)
T2    Tumour more than 2 cm but not more than 5 cm in greatest dimension (Fig. 267)
T3    Tumour more than 5 cm in greatest dimension (Fig. 267)
T4    Tumour of any size with direct extension to chest wall or skin, only as described in T4a to T4d

> **Note:**    Chest wall includes ribs, intercostal muscles and serratus anterior muscle but not pectoral muscle.

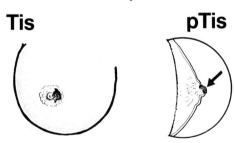

**Tis**          **pTis**

**Fig. 264**

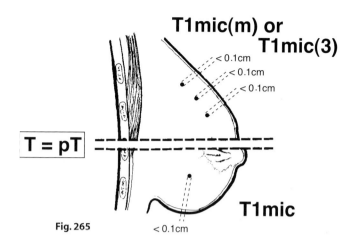

**T1mic(m) or T1mic(3)**

< 0.1cm
< 0.1cm
< 0.1cm

T = pT

**T1mic**

Fig. 265          < 0.1cm

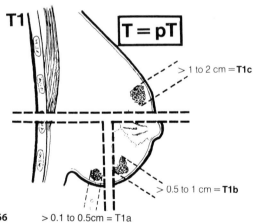

T1

T = pT

> 1 to 2 cm = **T1c**

> 0.5 to 1 cm = **T1b**

Fig. 266      > 0.1 to 0.5cm = T1a

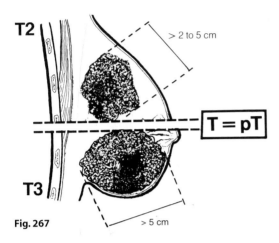

**T2**

> 2 to 5 cm

T = pT

**T3**

> 5 cm

**Fig. 267**

T4a   Extension to chest wall (Fig. 268)

T4b   Oedema (including peau d´orange), or ulceration of the skin of the breast, or satellite skin nodules confined to the same breast (Figs. 269, 270)

T4c   Both 4a and 4b above (Fig. 271)

T4d   Inflammatory carcinoma (Fig. 272)

**Notes:**   Inflammatory carcinoma of the breast is characterized by diffuse, brawny induration of the skin with an erysipeloid edge, usually with no underlying palpable mass. If the skin biopsy is negative and there is no localized measurable primary cancer, the T category is pTX when pathologically staging a clinical inflammatory carcinoma (T4d).

Dimpling of the skin, nipple retraction or other skin changes, except those in T4b and 4d, may occur in T1, T2 or T3 without affecting the classification.

# T4a     pT4a

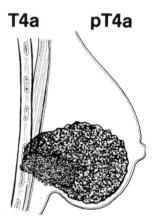

**Fig. 268**

# T4b           pT4b

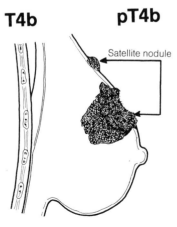

Satellite nodule

**Fig. 269**

**T4b**          **pT4b**

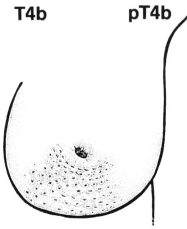

Fig. 270

**T4c**     **pT4c**

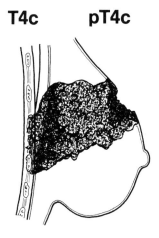

Fig. 271

**T4d**          **pT4d**

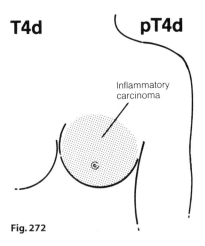

Inflammatory
carcinoma

Fig. 272

## N – Regional Lymph Nodes

NX    Regional lymph nodes cannot be assessed (e.g. previously removed)
N0    No regional lymph node metastasis
N1    Metastasis to movable ipsilateral axillary node(s) (Fig. 273)
N2    Metastasis to ipsilateral axillary node(s) fixed to one another or to other structures (Fig. 274)
N3    Metastasis to ipsilateral internal mammary lymph node(s) (Fig. 275)

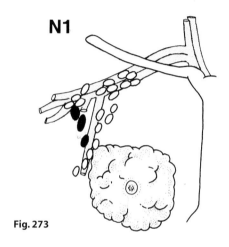

**Fig. 273**

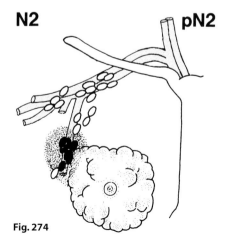

**Fig. 274**

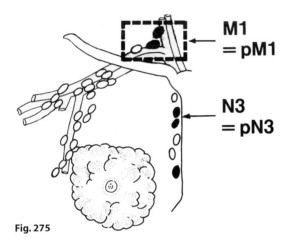

**Fig. 275**

## pTN Pathological Classification

### pT – Primary Tumour

The pathological classification requires the examination of the primary carcinoma with no gross tumour at the margins of resection. A case can be classified pT if there is only microscopic tumour in a margin.
The pT categories correspond to the T categories.

When classifying pT the tumour size is a measurement of the *invasive* component. If there is a large in situ component (e.g. 4 cm) and a small invasive component (e.g. 0.5 cm), the tumour is coded pT1a.

## pN – Regional Lymph Nodes

The pathological classification requires the resection and examination of at least the low axillary lymph nodes (level I) (see p. 203). Such a resection will ordinarily include 6 or more lymph nodes.

pNX  Regional lymph nodes cannot be assessed (not removed for study or previously removed)

pN0  No regional lymph node metastasis

pN1  Metastasis to movable ipsilateral axillary node(s)

    pN1a  Only micrometastasis (none larger than 0.2 cm) (Fig. 276)

    pN1b  Metastasis to lymph node(s), any larger than 0.2 cm (Fig. 277)

        pN1bi  Metastasis to one to three lymph nodes, any more than 0.2 cm and all less than 2.0 cm in greatest dimension

        pN1bii  Metastasis to four or more lymph nodes, any more than 0.2 cm and all less than 2.0 cm in greatest dimension

        pN1biii  Extension of tumour beyond the capsule of a lymph node metastasis less than 2.0 cm in greatest dimension

        pN1biv  Metastasis to a lymph node 2.0 cm or more in greatest dimension

pN2  Metastasis to ipsilateral axillary lymph nodes that are fixed to one another or to other structures (Fig. 274, see p. 209)

pN3  Metastasis to ipsilateral internal mammary lymph node(s) (Fig. 275, see p. 210)

## pN1a

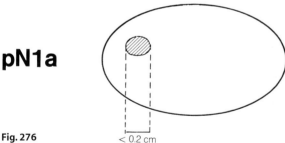

**Fig. 276**

< 0.2 cm

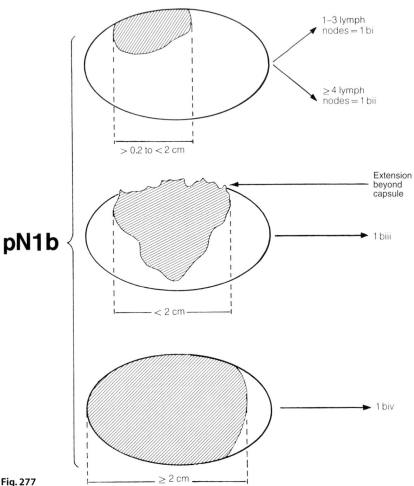

**pN1b**

1–3 lymph
nodes = 1 bi

≥ 4 lymph
nodes = 1 bii

> 0.2 to < 2 cm

Extension
beyond
capsule

1 biii

< 2 cm

1 biv

≥ 2 cm

**Fig. 277**

# Gynaecological Tumours

## Introductory Notes

The following sites are included:

Vulva
Vagina
Cervix uteri
Corpus uteri
Ovary
Fallopian tube
Gestational trophoblastic tumours

Cervix uteri and corpus uteri were amongst the first sites to be classified by the TNM system. The "League of Nations" stages for carcinoma of the cervix have been used with minor modifications for over 50 years, and, because these are accepted by the Fédération Internationale de Gynécologie et d´Obstétrique (FIGO), the TNM categories have been defined to correspond to the FIGO stages. Some amendments have been made in collaboration with FIGO, and the classifications now published have the approval of FIGO, UICC and the national TNM committees including AJCC.

# Vulva (ICD-O C51)

This classification is in complete agreement with the FIGO classification.

## Rules for Classification

The classification applies only to primary carcinomas of the vulva. There should be histological confirmation of the disease. A carcinoma of the vulva that has extended to the vagina is classified as carcinoma of the vulva.

The FIGO stages are based on surgical staging. (TNM stages are based on clinical and/or pathological classification.)

## Anatomical Subsites (Fig. 278)

1. Labia majora (C51.0)
2. Labia minora (C51.1)
3. Clitoris (C51.2)

## Regional Lymph Nodes

The regional lymph nodes are the femoral and inguinal nodes.

## TN Clinical Classification

### T – Primary Tumour

TX     Primary tumour cannot be assessed
T0     No evidence of primary tumour
Tis     Carcinoma in situ (preinvasive carcinoma)

T1    Tumour confined to vulva or vulva and perineum, 2 cm less in greatest dimension (Fig. 279)

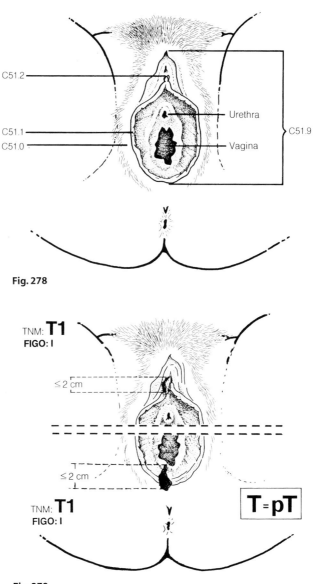

**Fig. 278**

**Fig. 279**

T1a    Tumour confined to vulva or vulva and perineum, 2 cm less in greatest dimension and with stromal invasion no greater than 1.0 mm (Fig. 280)

T1b    Tumour confined to vulva or vulva and perineum, 2 cm or less in greatest dimension and with stromal invasion greater than 1.0 mm (Fig. 280)

**Note:**    The depth of invasion is defined as the measurement of the tumour from the epithelial-stromal junction of the adjacent most superficial dermal papilla to the deepest point of invasion.

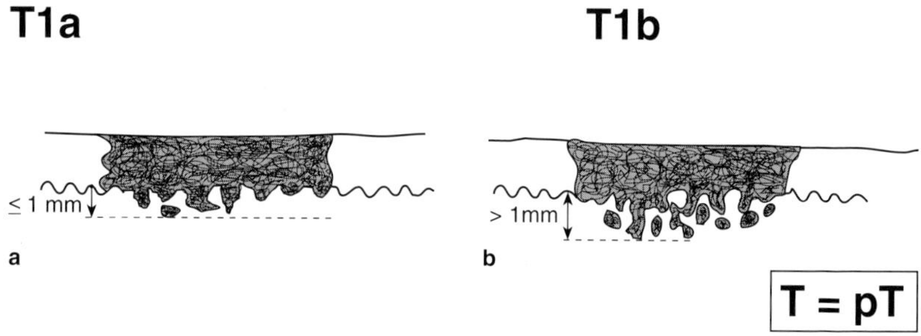

# T1a

# T1b

≤ 1 mm

> 1mm

a

b

T = pT

**Fig. 280a, b**

T2   Tumour confined to vulva or vulva and perineum, more than 2 cm in greatest dimension (Fig. 281)

T3   Tumour invades any of the following: lower urethra, vagina, anus (Figs. 282, 283)

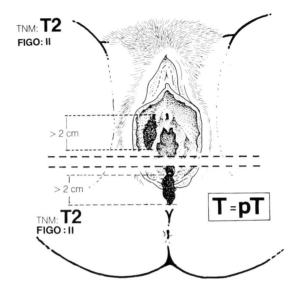

**Fig. 281**

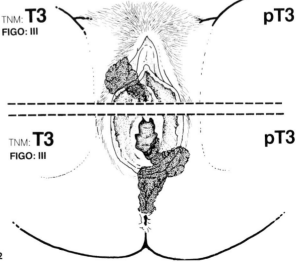

**Fig. 282**

T4    Tumour invades any of the following: bladder mucosa, rectal mucosa, upper urethral mucosa; or is fixed to bone (Fig. 284)

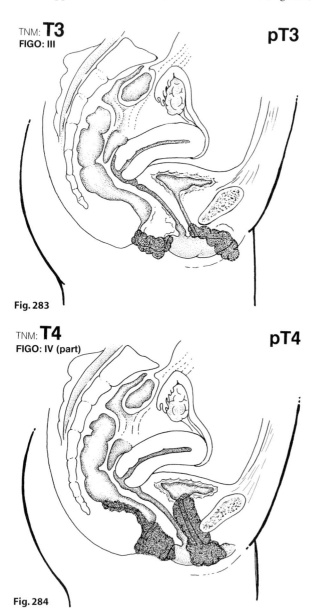

TNM: **T3**
**FIGO: III**

**pT3**

**Fig. 283**

TNM: **T4**
**FIGO: IV (part)**

**pT4**

**Fig. 284**

## N – Regional Lymph Nodes

NX    Regional lymph nodes cannot be assessed
N0    No regional lymph node metastasis
N1    Unilateral regional lymph node metastasis (Fig. 285)
N2    Bilateral regional lymph node metastasis (Fig. 286)

# pTN Pathological Classification

The pT and pN categories correspond to the T and N categories.

pN0    Histological examination of an inguinal lymphadenectomy specimen will ordinarily include 6 or more lymph nodes.

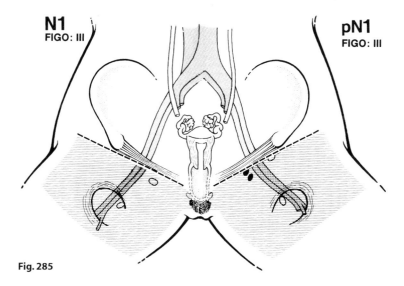

**N1**
FIGO: III

**pN1**
FIGO: III

**Fig. 285**

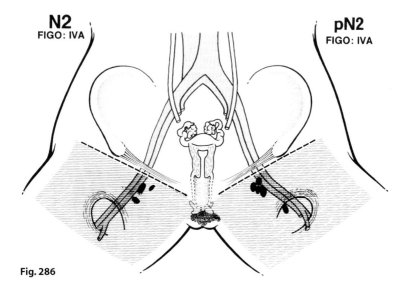

**N2**
FIGO: IVA

**pN2**
FIGO: IVA

**Fig. 286**

# Vagina (ICD-O C52) (Fig. 287)

The definitions of the T and M categories correspond to the FIGO stages. Both systems are included for comparison.

## Rules for Classification

The classification applies to primary carcinomas only.
Tumours present in the vagina as secondary growths from either genital or extragenital sites are excluded.
A tumour that has extended to the portio and reached the external os (orifice of uterus) is classified as carcinoma of the cervix.
A tumour involving the vulva is classified as carcinoma of the vulva.
There should be histological confirmation of the disease.

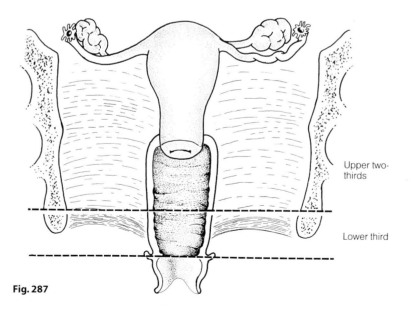

Upper two-thirds

Lower third

**Fig. 287**

## Regional Lymph Nodes

*Upper Two-Thirds of Vagina*
The pelvic nodes (Fig. 288)

*Lower Third of Vagina*
The inguinal nodes (Fig. 289)

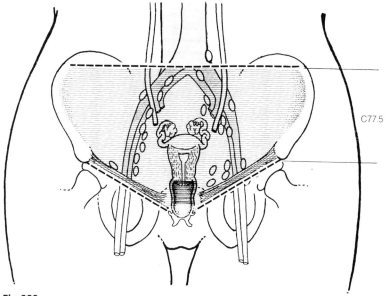

C77.5

**Fig. 288**

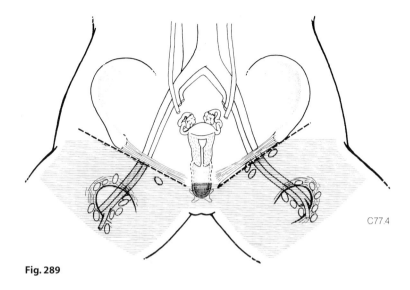

C77.4

**Fig. 289**

## TNM Clinical Classification

### T – Primary Tumour

| TNM categories | FIGO stages | |
|---|---|---|
| TX | | Primary tumour cannot be assessed |
| T0 | | No evidence of primary tumour |
| Tis | 0 | Carcinoma in situ |
| T1 | I | Tumour confined to vagina (Fig. 290) |
| T2 | II | Tumour invades paravaginal tissues but does not extend to pelvic wall (Fig. 291) |
| T3 | III | Tumour extends to pelvic wall (Fig. 292) |
| T4 | IVA | Tumour invades *mucosa* of bladder or rectum and/or extends beyond the true pelvis (Fig. 293) |
| | | **Note:** The presence of bullous oedema is not sufficient evidence to classify a tumour as T4. |
| M1 | IVB | Distant metastasis |

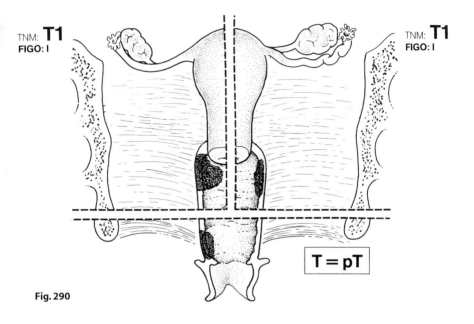

TNM: **T1**
FIGO: I

TNM: **T1**
FIGO: I

T = pT

**Fig. 290**

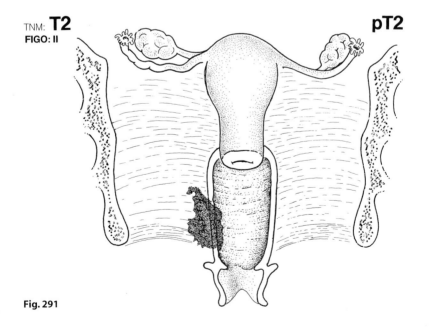

TNM: **T2**
FIGO: II

**pT2**

**Fig. 291**

TNM: **T3**
FIGO: III

**pT3**

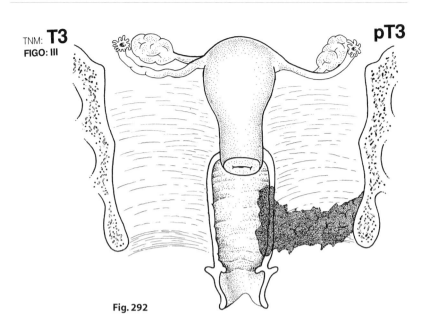

**Fig. 292**

TNM: **T4**
FIGO: IVA

**pT4**

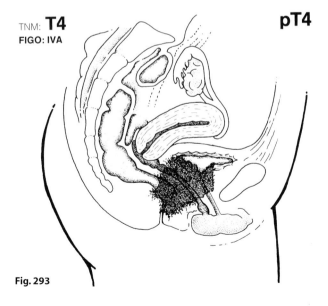

**Fig. 293**

## N – Regional Lymph Nodes

NX     Regional lymph nodes cannot be assessed
N0     No regional lymph node metastasis
N1     Pelvic or inguinal lymph node metastasis (Figs. 294-296)

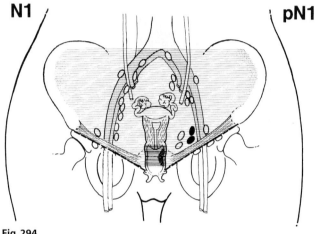

**Fig. 294**

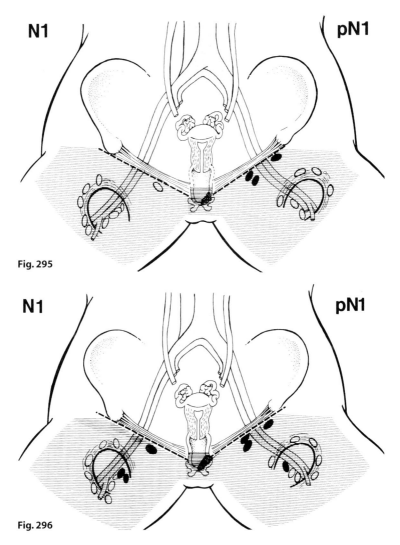

**N1**    **pN1**

Fig. 295

**N1**    **pN1**

Fig. 296

## pTN Pathological Classification

The pT and pN categories correspond to the T and N categories.

pN0    Histological examination of an inguinal lymphadenectomy specimen will ordinarily include 6 or more lymph nodes; a pelvic lymphadenectomy specimen will ordinarily include 10 or more lymph nodes.

# Cervix Uteri (ICD-O C53)

The definitions of the T and M categories correspond to the FIGO stages. Both systems are included for comparison.

## Rules for Classification

The classification applies only to carcinomas. There should be histological confirmation of the disease.

## Anatomical Subsites (Fig. 297)

1. Endocervix (C53.0)
2. Exocervix (C53.1)

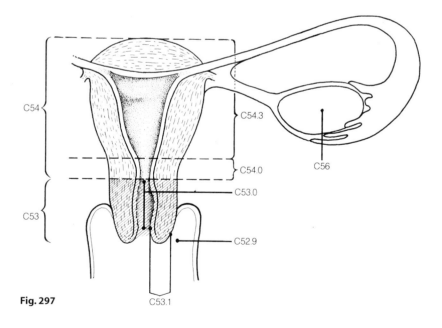

**Fig. 297**

## Regional Lymph Nodes (Fig. 298)

The regional lymph nodes are

*(1)* paracervical nodes
*(2)* parametrial nodes
*(3)* hypogastric (internal iliac) including obturator nodes
*(4)* external iliac nodes
*(5)* common iliac nodes
*(6)* presacral nodes
*(7)* lateral sacral nodes *(not shown in Fig. 298)*

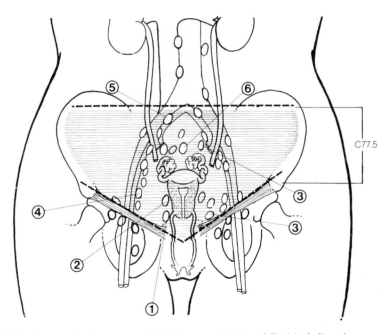

**Fig. 298.**   *1:* paracervical, *2:* parametrial, *3:* hypogastric (internal iliac) including obturator, *4:* external iliac, *5:* common iliac, *6:* presacral

# TNM Clinical Classification

## T – Primary Tumour

| TNM categories | FIGO stages | |
|---|---|---|
| TX | | Primary tumour cannot be assessed |
| T0 | | No evidence of primary tumour |
| Tis | 0 | Carcinoma in situ (preinvasive carcinoma) |
| T1 | I | Cervical carcinom confined to uterus (extension to corpus should be disregarded) |
| T1a | IA | Invasive carcinoma diagnosed only by microscopy. All macroscopically visible lesions – even with superficial invasion – are T1b/Stage IB (Fig. 299) |
| T1a1 | IA1 | Stromal invasion no greater than 3.0 mm in depth and 7.0 mm or less in horizontal spread (Fig. 300) |
| T1a2 | IA2 | Stromal invasion more than 3.0 mm and not more than 5.0 mm with a horizontal spread 7.0 mm or less (Fig. 301) |
| | | **Note:** The depth of invasion should not be more than 5 mm taken from the base of the epithelium, either surface or glandular, from which it originates. The depth of invasion is defined as the measurement of the tumour from the epithelial-stromal junction of the adjacent most superficial epithelial papilla to the deepest point of invasion. Vascular space involvement. venous or lymphatic, does not affect classification |
| T1b | IB | Clinically visible lesion confined to the cervix (Figs. 302, 304) or microscopic lesion greater than T1a2/IA2 (Fig. 303) |
| T1b1 | IB1 | Clinically visible lesion 4.0 cm or less in greatest dimension (Fig. 302) |
| T1b2 | IB2 | Clinically visible lesion more than 4 cm in greatest dimension (Fig. 304) |
| T2 | II | Tumour invades beyond uterus but not to pelvic wall or to lower third of the vagina (Fig. 305) |
| T2a | IIA | Without parametrial invasion |
| T2b | IIB | With parametrial invasion |

TNM: **T1a**    **pT1a**
FIGO: **IA**

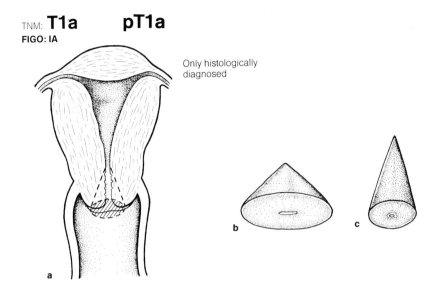

Only histologically
diagnosed

**Fig. 299a–c**

TNM: **T1a1**    **pT1a1**

FIGO: **IA1**

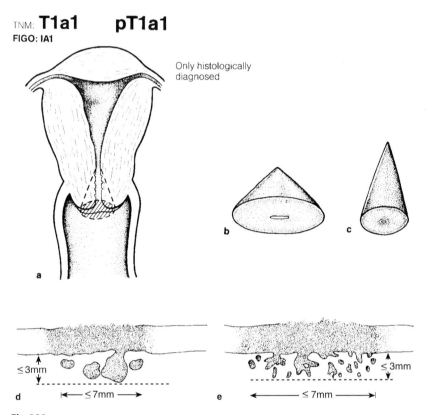

Only histologically
diagnosed

**Fig. 300a–e**

TNM: **T1a2**    **pT1a2**
FIGO: IA 2

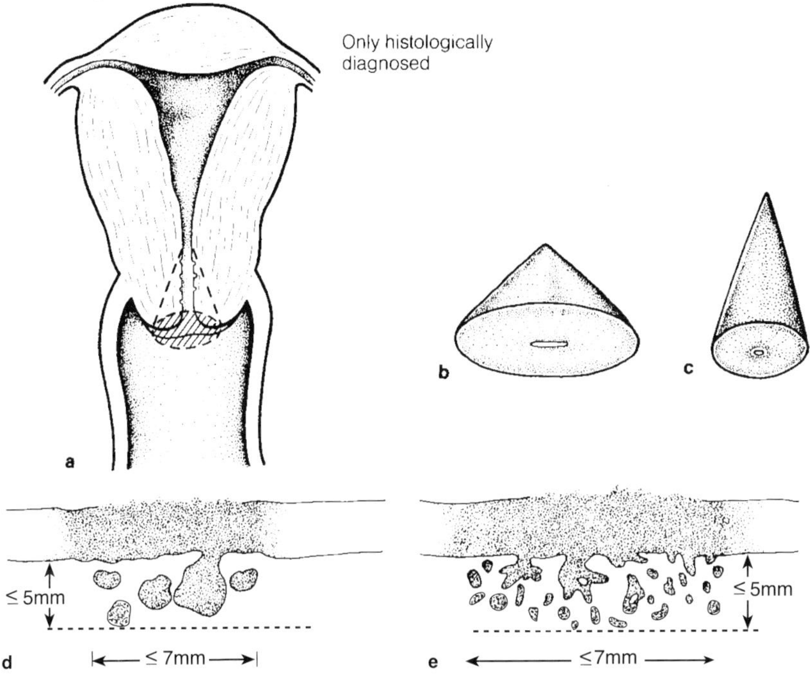

Only histologically
diagnosed

≤ 5mm

a

b

c

d   |← ≤ 7mm →|

e   ← ≤7mm →

≤5mm

**Fig. 301a–e**

TNM: **T1b1**    **pT1b1**
FIGO: IB1

**Fig. 302**   ≤4cm

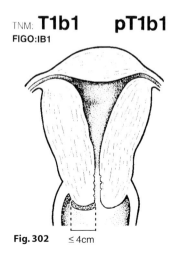

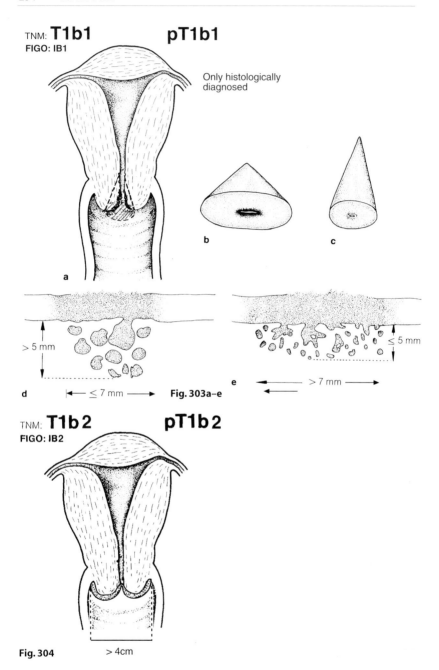

TNM: **T1b1**    **pT1b1**
FIGO: IB1

Only histologically
diagnosed

b

c

a

> 5 mm

≤ 7 mm

d

**Fig. 303a–e**

≤ 5 mm

> 7 mm

e

TNM: **T1b2**    **pT1b2**
FIGO: IB2

**Fig. 304**

> 4cm

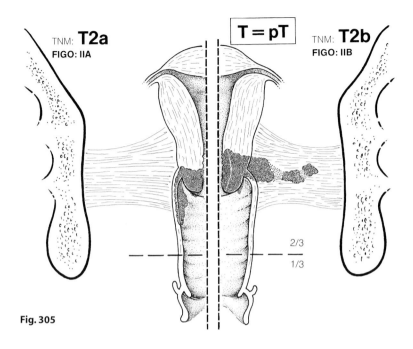

2/3
1/3

**Fig. 305**

| TNM categories | FIGO stages | |
|---|---|---|
| T3 | III | Tumour extends to pelvic wall and/or involves the lower third of vagina and/or causes hydronephrosis or non-functioning kidney (Fig. 306) |
| T3a | IIIA | Tumour involves lower third of vagina, no extension to pelvic wall |
| T3b | IIIB | Tumour extends to pelvic wall and/or causes hydronephrosis or non-functioning kidney |
| T4 | IVA | Tumour invades *mucosa* of bladder or rectum and/or extends beyond true pelvis (Fig. 307) |
| | | **Note:** The presence of bullous oedema is not sufficient evidence to classify a tumour as T4. |
| M1 | IVB | Distant metastasis |

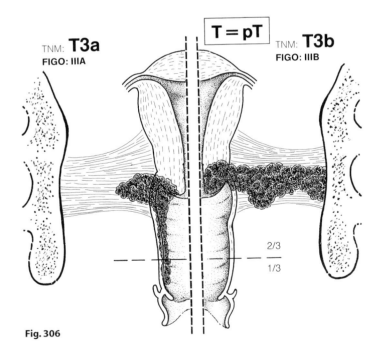

TNM: **T3a**
FIGO: **IIIA**

T = pT

TNM: **T3b**
FIGO: **IIIB**

2/3

1/3

**Fig. 306**

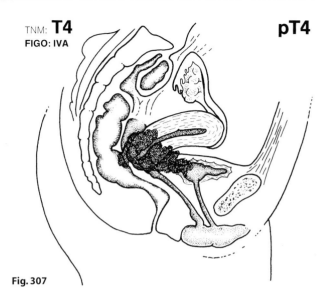

TNM: **T4**
FIGO: IVA

**pT4**

**Fig. 307**

## N – Regional Lymph Nodes

NX     Regional lymph nodes cannot be assessed
N0     No regional lymph node metastasis
N1     Regional lymph node metastasis (Fig. 308)

## pTN Pathological Classification

The pT and pN categories correspond to the T and N categories.

pN0    Histological examination of a pelvic lymphadenectomy specimen will ordinarily include 10 or more lymph nodes.

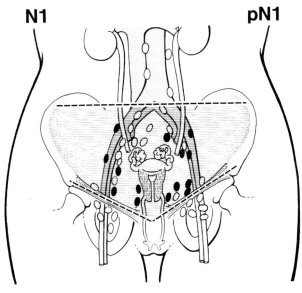

**N1**                                                    **pN1**

**Fig. 308**

# Corpus Uteri (ICD-O C54)

The definitions of the T, N and M categories correspond to the FIGO stages. Both systems are included for comparison.

## Rules for Classification

The classification applies only to carcinomas. There should be histological verification and grading of the tumour. The diagnosis should be based on examination of specimens taken by endometrial biopsy.

The FIGO stages are based on surgical staging. (TNM stages are based on clinical and/or pathological classification).

## Anatomical Subsites (See Fig. 297, p. 228)

1. Isthmus uteri (C54.0)
2. Fundus uteri (C54.3)

## Regional Lymph Nodes (See Fig. 314, p. 245)

The regional lymph nodes are:
1. The pelvic nodes
 – hypogastric (internal iliac) including obturator nodes (1)
 – common iliac nodes (2)
 – external iliac nodes (3)
 – parametrial nodes (not shown)
 – sacral nodes (4)
and
2. The para-aortic nodes (5)

# TNM Clinical Classification

## T – Primary Tumour

| TNM categories | FIGO stages | |
|---|---|---|
| TX | | Primary tumour cannot be assessed |
| T0 | | No evidence of primary tumour |
| Tis | 0 | Carcinoma in situ (preinvasive carcinoma) |
| T1 | I | Tumour confined to corpus uteri (Fig. 309) |
| T1a | IA | Tumour limited to endometrium |
| T1b | IB | Tumour invades up to or less than one half of myometrium |
| T1c | IC | Tumour invades more than one half of myometrium |
| T2 | II | Tumour invades cervix but does not extend beyond uterus (Fig. 310) |
| T2a | IIA | Endocervical glandular involvement only |
| T2b | IIB | Cervical stromal invasion |
| T3 and/or N1 | III | Local and/or regional spread as specified in T3a, b, N1 and FIGO IIIA, B, C below |
| T3a | IIIA | Tumour involves serosa and/or adnexa (direct extension or metastasis) and/or cancer cells in ascites or peritoneal washings (Fig. 311) |
| T3b | IIIB | Vaginal involvement (direct extension or metastasis) (Fig. 311) |
| N1 | IIIC | Metastasis to pelvic and/or para-aortic lymph nodes (Fig. 313) |
| T4 | IVA | Tumour invades bladder *mucosa* and/or bowel *mucosa* (Fig. 312) |
| M1 | IVB | Distant metastasis (*excluding* metastasis to vagina, pelvic serosa or adnexa, *including* metastasis to intra-abdominal lymph nodes other than para-aortic and/or inguina lymph nodes) |

**Note:**   The presence of bullous edema is not sufficient evidence to classify a tumour as T4.

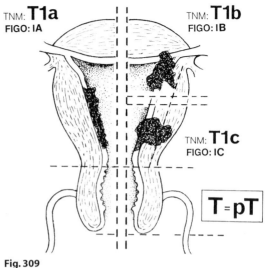

TNM: **T1a**
FIGO: IA

TNM: **T1b**
FIGO: IB

TNM: **T1c**
FIGO: IC

T = pT

**Fig. 309**

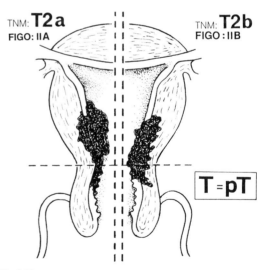

TNM: **T2a**
FIGO: IIA

TNM: **T2b**
FIGO: IIB

T = pT

**Fig. 310**

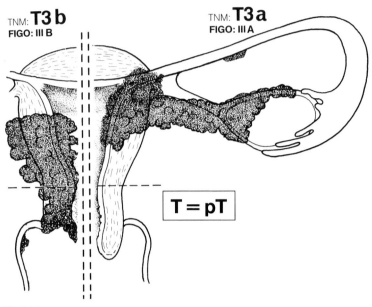

TNM: **T3 b**
FIGO: III B

TNM: **T3 a**
FIGO: III A

T = pT

**Fig. 311**

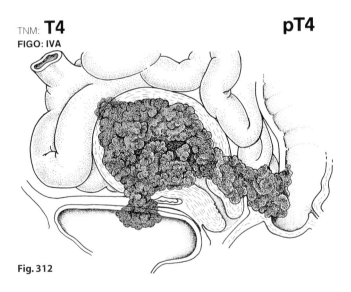

TNM: **T4**
FIGO: IVA

**pT4**

**Fig. 312**

## N – Regional Lymph Nodes

NX     Regional lymph nodes cannot be assessed
N0     No regional lymph node metastasis
N1     Regional lymph node metastasis (Fig. 313)

# pTN Pathological Classification

The pT and pN categories correspond to the T and N categories.

pN0     Histological examination of a pelvic lymphadenectomy specimen will
         ordinarily include 10 or more lymph nodes.

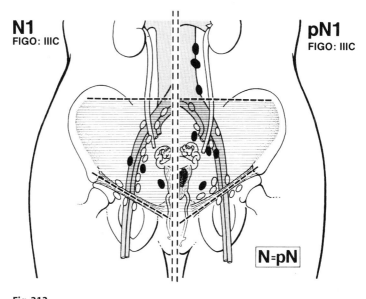

**Fig. 313**

# Ovary (ICD-O C56) (See Fig. 297, p. 228)

The definitions of the T, N and M categories correspond to the FIGO stages. Both systems are included for comparison.

## Rules for Classification

There should be histological confirmation of the disease and division of cases by histological type. In accordance with FIGO, a simplified version of the WHO histological classification of common epithielial tumours (International Histological Clas-sification of Tumours No. 9, WHO, Geneva 1973) is recommended. The degree of differentiation (grade) should be recorded.

## Regional Lymph Nodes (Fig. 314)

The regional nodes are

*(1)* hypogastric (internal iliac) including obturator nodes
*(2)* common iliac nodes
*(3)* external iliac nodes
*(4)* lateral sacral nodes
*(5)* para-aortic nodes
*(6)* inguinal nodes

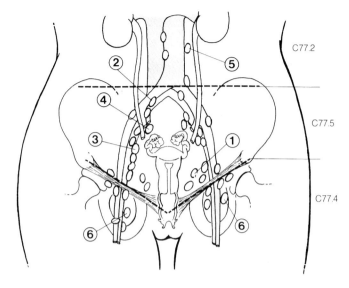

**Fig. 314.** *1* hypogastric; *2* common iliac; *3* external iliac; *4* lateral sacral; *5* para-aortic; *6* inguinal

## TNM Clinical Classification

### T – Primary Tumour

| TNM categories | FIGO stages | |
|---|---|---|
| TX | | Primary tumour cannot be assessed |
| T0 | | No evidence of primary tumour |
| T1 | I | Tumour limited to ovaries |
| T1a | IA | Tumour limited to one ovary; capsule intact, no tumour on ovarian surface; no malignant cells in ascites or peritoneal washings (Fig. 315) |
| T1b | IB | Tumour limited to both ovaries; capsules intact, no tumour on ovarian surface: no malignant cells in ascites or peritoneal washings (Fig. 316) |

| TNM categories | FIGO stages | |
|---|---|---|
| T1c | IC | Tumour limited to one or both ovaries with any of the following: capsule ruptured, tumour on ovarian surface, malignant cells in ascites or peritoneal washings (Fig. 317) |
| T2 | II | Tumour involves one or both ovaries with pelvic extension |
| T2a | IIA | Extension and/or implants on uterus and/or tube(s); no malignant cells in ascites or peritoneal washings (Fig. 318) |
| T2b | IIB | Extension to other pelvic tissues; no malignant cells in ascites or peritoneal washings (Fig. 319) |
| T2c | IIC | Pelvic extension (2a or 2b) with malignant cells in ascites or peritoneal washings (Fig. 320) |
| T3 and/or N1 | III | Tumour involves one or both ovaries with microscopically confirmed peritoneal metastasis outside the pelvis and/or regional lymph node metastasis (Figs. 321–323) |
| T3a | IIIA | Microscopic peritoneal metastasis beyond pelvis |
| T3b | IIIB | Macroscopic peritoneal metastasis beyond pelvis 2 cm or less in greatest dimension |
| T3c and/ or N1 | IIIC | Peritoneal metastasis beyond pelvis more than 2 cm in greatest dimension and/or regional lymph node metastasis (Fig. 323) |
| M1 | IV | Distant metastasis (excludes peritoneal metastasis) (Fig. 322) |

**Note:** Liver capsule metastasis is T3/stage III, liver parenchymal metastasis M1/stage IV. Pleural effusion must have positive cytology for M1/stage IV (Fig. 322).

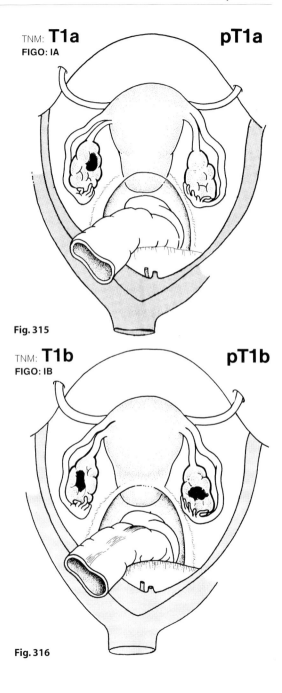

TNM: **T1a**
FIGO: IA

**pT1a**

Fig. 315

TNM: **T1b**
FIGO: IB

**pT1b**

Fig. 316

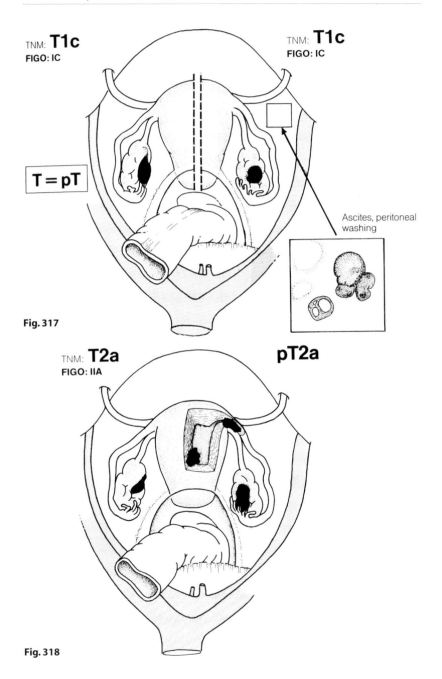

TNM: **T1c**
FIGO: IC

TNM: **T1c**
FIGO: IC

T = pT

Ascites, peritoneal
washing

**Fig. 317**

TNM: **T2a**
FIGO: IIA

**pT2a**

**Fig. 318**

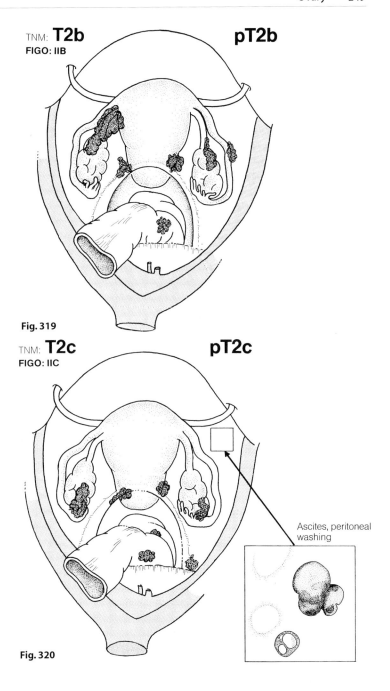

TNM: **T2b**
FIGO: IIB

**pT2b**

Fig. 319

TNM: **T2c**
FIGO: IIC

**pT2c**

Ascites, peritoneal washing

Fig. 320

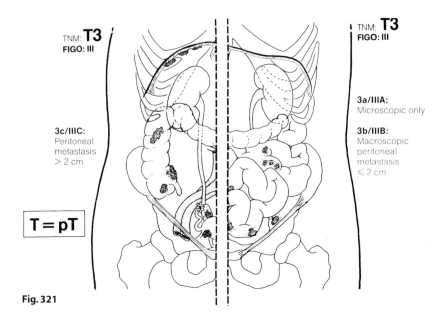

TNM: **T3**
FIGO: III

TNM: **T3**
FIGO: III

**3a/IIIA:**
Microscopic only

**3b/IIIB:**
Macroscopic
peritoneal
metastasis
≤ 2 cm

**3c/IIIC:**
Peritoneal
metastasis
> 2 cm

$T = pT$

**Fig. 321**

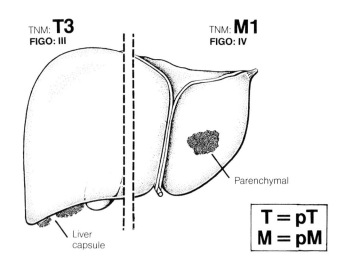

TNM: **T3**
FIGO: III

TNM: **M1**
FIGO: IV

Parenchymal

Liver
capsule

$T = pT$
$M = pM$

**Fig. 322**

## N – Regional Lymph Nodes

NX    Regional lymph nodes cannot be assessed
N0    No regional lymph node metastasis
N1    Regional lymph node metastasis (Fig. 323)

**N1**                                                    **pN1**

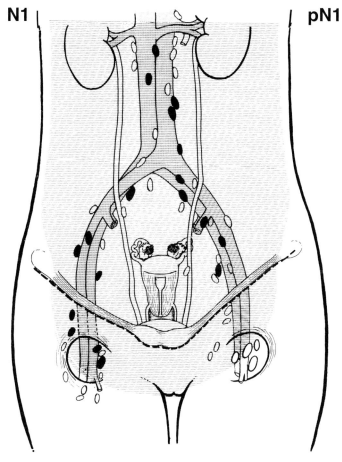

**Fig. 323**

### M – Distant Metastasis

MX    Distant metastasis cannot be assessed
M0    No distant metastasis
M1    Distant metastasis (Fig. 322)

## pTNM Pathological Classification

The pT, pN and pM categories correspond to the T, N and M categories.

pN0    Histological examination of a pelvic lymphadenectomy specimen will ordinarily include 10 or more lymph nodes.

# Fallopian Tube (ICD-O C57.0)

The following classification for carcinoma of the fallopian tube is based on that of FIGO adopted in 1992. The definitions of the T, N and M categories correspond to the FIGO stages. Both systems are included for comparison.

## Rules for Classification

The classification applies only to carcinoma. There should be histological confirmation of the disease.
The FIGO stages are based on surgical staging. (TNM stages are based on clinical and/or pathological staging.)

## Regional Lymph Nodes

The regional lymph nodes are the hypogastric (obturator), common iliac, external iliac, lateral sacral, para-aortic and inguinal nodes (see Fig. 314, p. 245).

## TNM Clinical Classification

### T – Primary Tumour

| TNM Categories | FIGO Stages | |
|---|---|---|
| TX | | Primary tumour cannot be assessed |
| T0 | | No evidence of primary tumour |
| Tis | 0 | Carcinoma in situ (preinvasive carcinoma) |
| T1 | I | Tumour confined to fallopian tube(s) |
| T1a | IA | Tumour limited to one tube, without penetrating the serosal surface; no ascites (Fig. 324) |
| T1b | IB | Tumour limited to both tubes, without penetrating the serosal surface; no ascites (Fig. 325) |

| TNM Categories | FIGO Stages | |
|---|---|---|
| T1c | IC | Tumour limited to one or both tube(s) with extension onto or through the tubal serosa, or with malignant cells in ascites or peritoneal washings (Fig. 326) |
| T2 | II | Tumour involves one or both fallopian tube(s) with pelvic extension |
| T2a | IIA | Extension and/or metastasis to uterus and/or ovaries (Fig. 327) |
| T2b | IIB | Extension to other pelvic structures (Fig. 328) |
| T2c | IIC | Pelvic extension (2a or 2b) with malignant cells in ascites or peritoneal washings (Fig. 329) |
| T3 and/or N1 | III | Tumour involves one or both fallopian tube(s) with peritoneal implants outside the pelvis and/or positive regional lymph nodes (Figs. 321–323, pp. 250–251) |
| T3a | IIIA | Microscopic peritoneal metastasis outside the pelvis |
| T3b | IIIB | Macroscopic peritoneal metastasis outside the pelvis 2 cm or less in greatest dimension |
| T3c and/ or N1 | IIIC | Peritoneal metastasis more than 2 cm in greatest dimension and/or positive regional lymph nodes (see Fig. 323, p. 251) |
| M1 | IV | Distant metastasis (excludes peritoneal metastasis) (see Fig. 322, p. 250) |

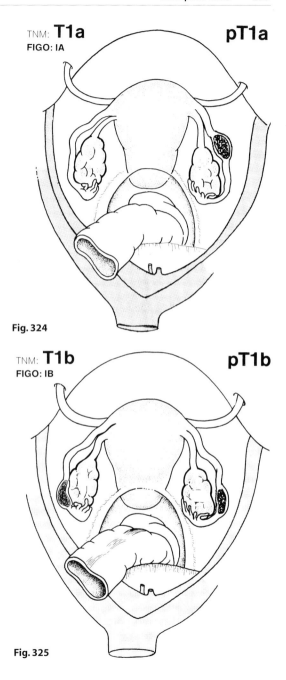

TNM: **T1a**
FIGO: IA

**pT1a**

**Fig. 324**

TNM: **T1b**
FIGO: IB

**pT1b**

**Fig. 325**

TNM: **T1c**
FIGO: IC

**pT1c**

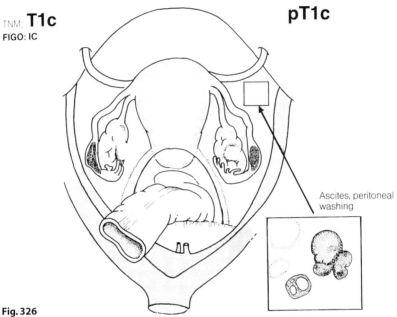

Ascites, peritoneal washing

**Fig. 326**

TNM: **T2a**
FIGO: IIA

**pT2a**

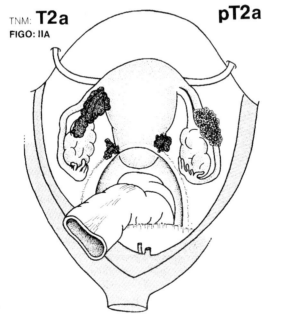

**Fig. 327**

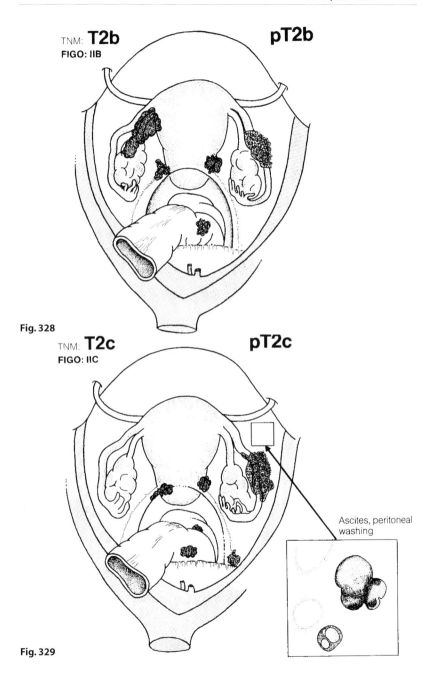

TNM: **T2b**
FIGO: **IIB**

**pT2b**

**Fig. 328**

TNM: **T2c**
FIGO: **IIC**

**pT2c**

Ascites, peritoneal washing

**Fig. 329**

## N – Regional Lymph Nodes

NX    Regional lymph nodes cannot be assessed
N0    No regional lymph node metastasis
N1    Regional lymph node metastasis

## M – Distant Metastasis

MX    Distant metastasis cannot be assessed
M0    No distant metastasis
M1    Distant metastasis

# pTNM Pathological Classification

The pT, pN and pM categories correspond to the T, N and M categories.

pN0   Histological examination of a pelvic lymphadenectomy specimen will
      ordinarily include 10 or more lymph nodes.

# Gestational Trophoblastic Tumours (ICD-O C58.9)

The following classification for gestational trophoblastic tumours is based on that of FIGO adopted in 1992. The definitions of T and M categories correspond to the FIGO stages. Both systems are included for comparison. In stage grouping, risk factors are considered in addition to T and M. In contrast to other sites, an N (regional lymph node) classification does not apply to these tumours.

## Rules for Classification

The classification applies to choriocarcinoma (9100/3), invasive hydatidiform mole (9100/1) and placental site trophoblastic tumour (9104/1). Placental site tumours should be reported separately. Histological confirmation is not required if the urine human chorionic gonadotropin (hCG) level is abnormally elevated. History of prior chemotherapy for this disease should be noted.

# TM Clinical Classification

## T – Primary Tumour

| TM Categories | FIGO Stages | |
|---|---|---|
| TX | | Primary tumour cannot he assessed |
| T0 | | No evidence of primary tumour |
| T1 | I | Tumour confined to uterus (Fig. 330) |
| T2 | II | Tumour extends to other genital structures: vagina, ovary, broad ligament, fallopian tube by metastasis or direct extension (Fig. 331) |
| M1a | III | Metastasis to the lung(s) |
| M1b | IV | Other distant metastasis with or without lung involvement |

**Note:** Stages I to IV are subdivided into A to C according to the number of risk factors:
A   without risk factors
B   with one risk factor
C   with two risk factors

**Risk factors:**    There are two major risk factors that may affect outcome (other than T and M):
1. hCG more than 100 000 IU/24 h urine
2. Detection of disease longer than 6 months from termination of antecedent pregnancy

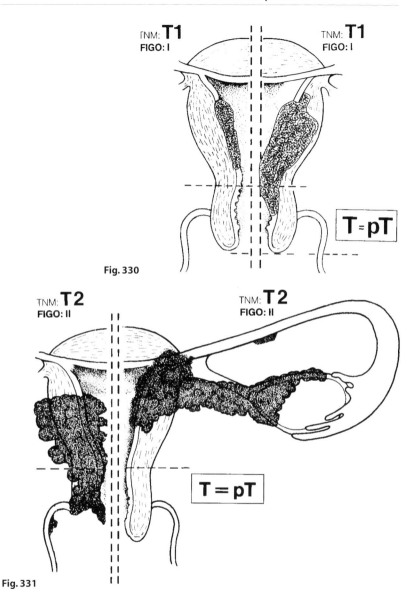

Fig. 330

Fig. 331

## pTM Pathological Classification

The pT and pM categories correspond to the T and M categories.

# Urological Tumours

## Introductory Notes

The following sites are included:

Penis
Prostate
Testis
Kidney
Renal pelvis and ureter
Urinary bladder
Urethra

# Penis (ICD-O C60)

## Rules for Classification

The classification applies only to carcinomas. There should be histological confirmation of the disease.

## Anatomical Subsites (Fig. 332)

1. Prepuce (C60.0)
2. Glans penis (C60.1)
3. Shaft of penis (C60.2)

## Regional Lymph Nodes

The regional lymph nodes are the superficial and deep inguinal and the pelvic nodes.

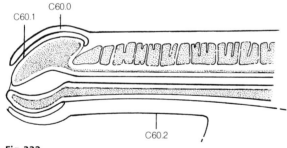

**Fig. 332**

# TN Clinical Classification

## T – Primary Tumour

TX    Primary tumour cannot be assessed
T0    No evidence of primary tumour
Tis   Carcinoma in situ
Ta    Non-invasive verrucous carcinoma (Fig. 333)

T1    Tumour invades subepithelial connective tissue (Fig. 334)
T2    Tumour invades corpus spongiosum or cavernosum (Fig. 335)
T3    Tumour invades urethra (Fig. 336) or prostate (Fig. 337)
T4    Tumour invades other adjacent structures (Figs. 338, 339)

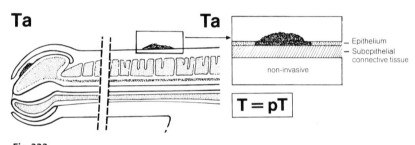

**Fig. 333**

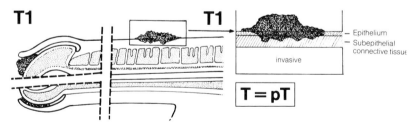

**Fig. 334**

**T2**                                        **T2**

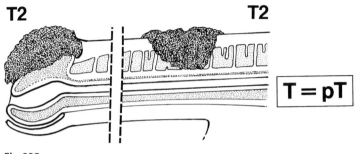

$\boxed{T = pT}$

Fig. 335

**T3**                                        **T3**

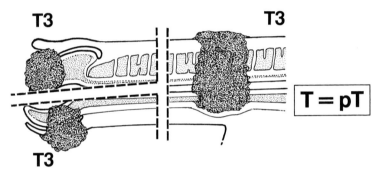

$\boxed{T = pT}$

**T3**

Fig. 336

**T3**                **pT3**

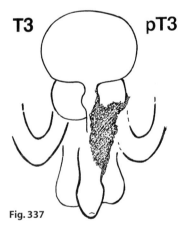

Fig. 337

**T4**    **pT4**

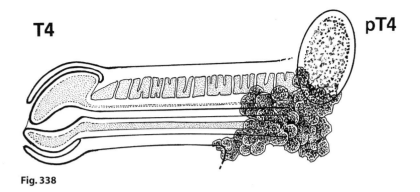

**Fig. 338**

**T4**    **pT4**

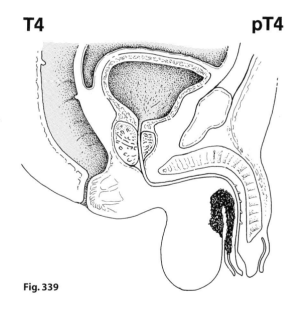

**Fig. 339**

## N – Regional Lymph Nodes

NX    Regional lymph nodes cannot be assessed
N0    No regional lymph node metastasis
N1    Metastasis in a single superficial inguinal lymph node (Fig. 340)

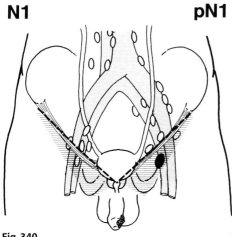

**Fig. 340**

N2    Metastasis in multiple (Fig. 341) or bilateral superficial inguinal lymph
       nodes (Fig. 342)

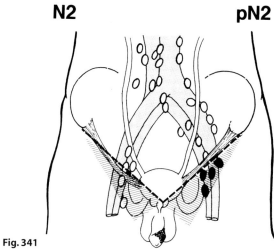

**Fig. 341**

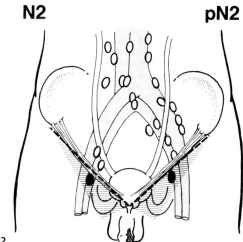

**Fig. 342**

N3    Metastasis in deep inguinal (Fig. 343) or pelvic lymph node(s), unilateral
(Fig. 344) or bilateral (Fig. 345)

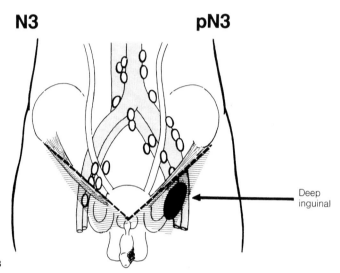

**Fig. 343**

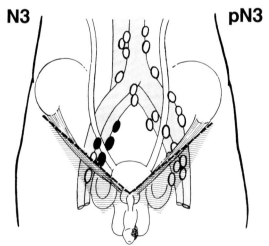

**Fig. 344**

**N3**

**pN3**

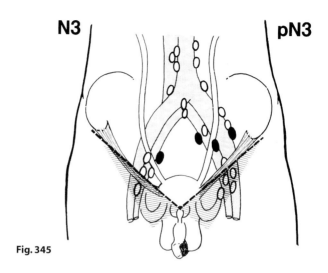

Fig. 345

## pTN Pathological Classification

The pT and pN categories correspond to the T and N categories.

# Prostate (ICD-O C61) [Figs. 346, 397 (see p. 309)]

## Rules for Classification

The classification applies only to adenocarcinomas. Transitional cell carcinoma of the prostate is classified as a urethral tumour (see pp. 315 and 320 ff.). There should be histological confirmation of the disease.

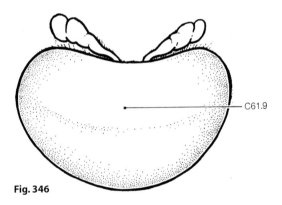

C61.9

**Fig. 346**

## Regional Lymph Nodes (Fig. 347)

The regional lymph nodes are the nodes of the true pelvis, which essentially are the pelvic nodes below the bifurcation of the common iliac arteries. Laterality does not affect the N classification.

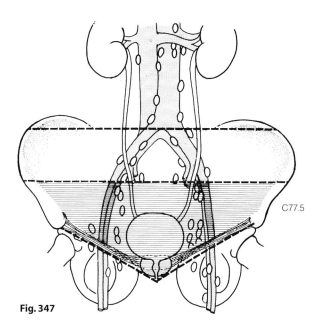

C77.5

**Fig. 347**

## TN Clinical Classification

### T – Primary Tumour

TX     Primary tumour cannot be assessed
T0     No evidence of primary tumour

T1     Clinically inapparent tumour not palpable nor visible by imaging
       (Fig. 348)
       T1a     Tumour incidental finding in 5% or less of tissue resected
       T1b     Tumour incidental finding in more than 5% of tissue resected
       T1c     Tumour identified by needle biopsy (e.g. because of elevated PSA)
T2     Tumour confined within prostate
       T2a     Tumour involves one lobe (Fig. 349)
       T2b     Tumour involves both lobes (Fig. 350)

> **Note:** Tumour found in one or both lobes by needle biopsy, but not palpable or
> visible by imaging is classified as T1c.

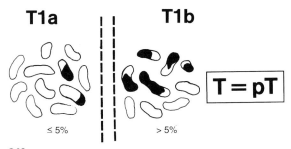

**Fig. 348**

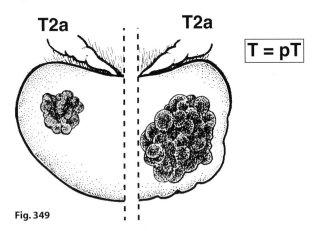

**Fig. 349**

T3    Tumour extends through prostatic capsule
   T3a   Extracapsular extension (unilateral or bilateral) (Fig. 351, 352)
   T3b   Tumour invades seminal vesicle(s) (Fig. 353)

   **Note:** Invasion into the prostatic apex or into (but not beyond) the prostatic
   capsule is not classified as T3, but as T2.

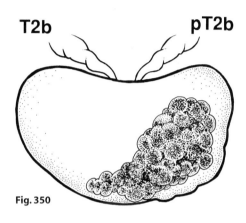

**T2b**                                    **pT2b**

Fig. 350

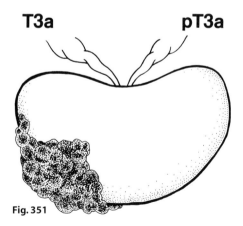

**T3a**                                    **pT3a**

Fig. 351

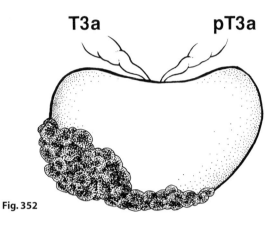

**Fig. 352**

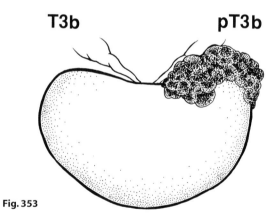

**Fig. 353**

T4    Tumour is fixed or invades adjacent structures other than seminal vesic-
les: bladder neck, external sphincter, rectum, levator muscles, and/or pelvic wall (Figs. 354, 355)

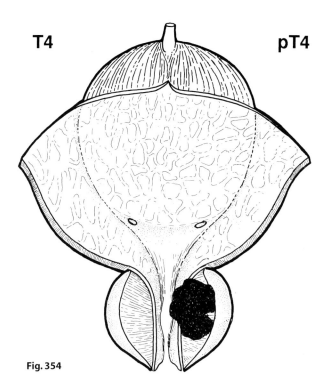

**T4**                                                                    **pT4**

**Fig. 354**

**T4**    **pT4**

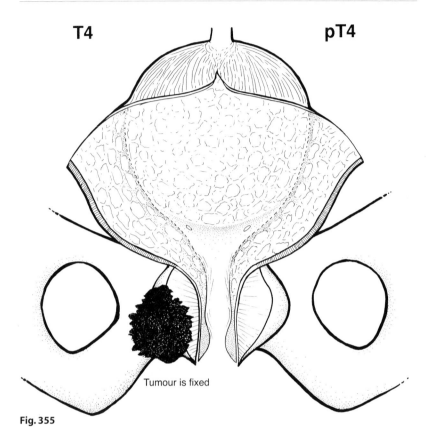

Tumour is fixed

**Fig. 355**

## N – Regional Lymph Nodes

NX    Regional lymph nodes cannot be assessed
N0    No regional lymph node metastasis
N1    Regional lymph node metastasis (Figs. 356, 357)

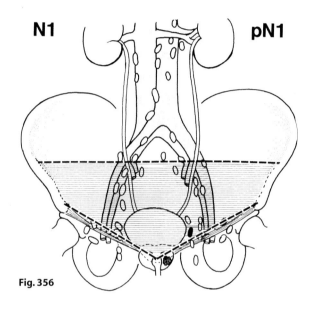

**Fig. 356**

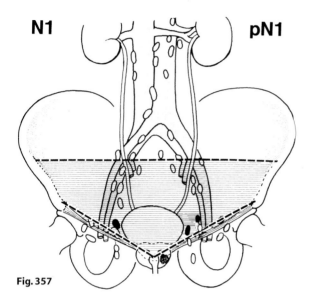

**N1**                    **pN1**

**Fig. 357**

## pTN Pathological Classification

The pT and pN categories correspond to the T and N categories.
However, there is no pT1 category because there is insufficient tissue to assess
the highest pT category.

# Testis (ICD-O C62) (Fig. 358)

## Rules for Classification

The classification applies only to germ cell tumours of the testis. There should be histological confirmation of the disease and division of cases by histological type. Histopathological grading is not applicable.

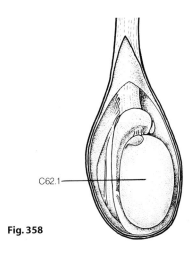

C62.1

**Fig. 358**

## Regional Lymph Nodes (Fig. 359)

The regional lymph nodes are the abdominal para-aortic (periaortic), preaortic, interaortocaval, precaval, paracaval, retrocaval and retroaortic nodes. Nodes along the spermatic vein should be considered regional. Laterality does not affect the N classification. The intrapelvic nodes and the inguinal nodes are considered regional after scrotal or inguinal surgery.

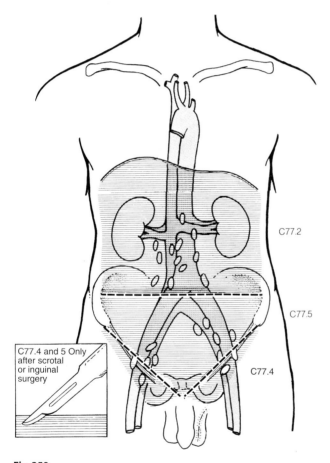

C77.2

C77.5

C77.4 and 5 Only
after scrotal
or inguinal
surgery

C77.4

**Fig. 359**

# TN Clinical Classification

## T – Primary Tumour

The extent of primary tumour is classified after radical orchiectomy, see pT. If no radical orchiectomy has been performed, TX is used.

## N – Regional Lymph Nodes

NX   Regional lymph nodes cannot be assessed
N0   No regional lymph node metastasis
N1   Metastasis with a lymph node mass 2 cm or less in greatest dimension (Figs. 360, 362, 365) or multiple lymph nodes, none more than 2 cm in greatest dimension (Figs. 361, 363, 364)
N2   Metastasis with a lymph node mass more than 2 cm but not more than 5 cm in greatest dimension (Figs. 366, 368) or multiple lymph nodes, any one mass more than 2 cm but not more than 5 cm in greatest dimension (Fig. 367)
N3   Metastasis with a lymph node mass more than 5 cm in greatest dimension (Figs. 369–372)

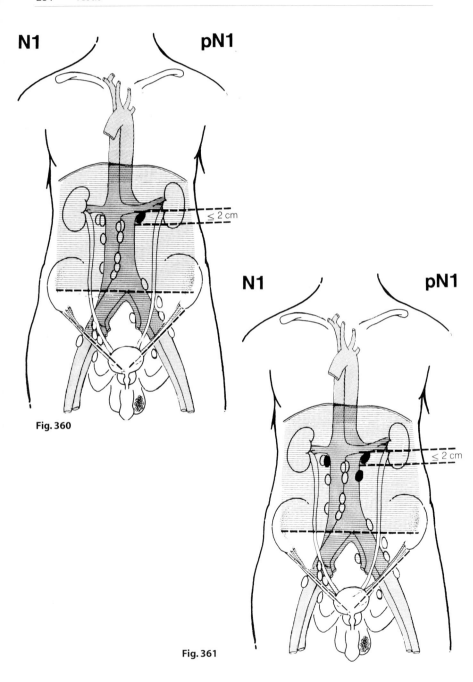

**N1** **pN1**

≤ 2 cm

**Fig. 360**

**N1** **pN1**

≤ 2 cm

**Fig. 361**

**N1**          **pN1**

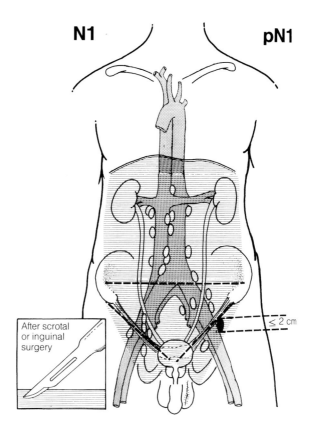

After scrotal
or inguinal
surgery

≤ 2 cm

**Fig. 362**

**N1**                                          **pN1**

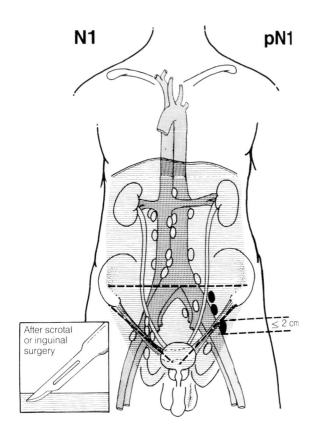

After scrotal
or inguinal
surgery

≤ 2 cm

**Fig. 363**

**N1**    **pN2**

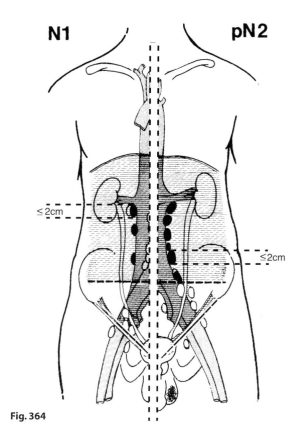

≤2cm

≤2cm

**Fig. 364**

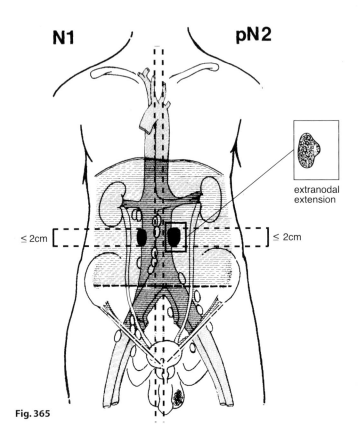

**N1**  **pN2**

extranodal
extension

≤ 2cm    ≤ 2cm

**Fig. 365**

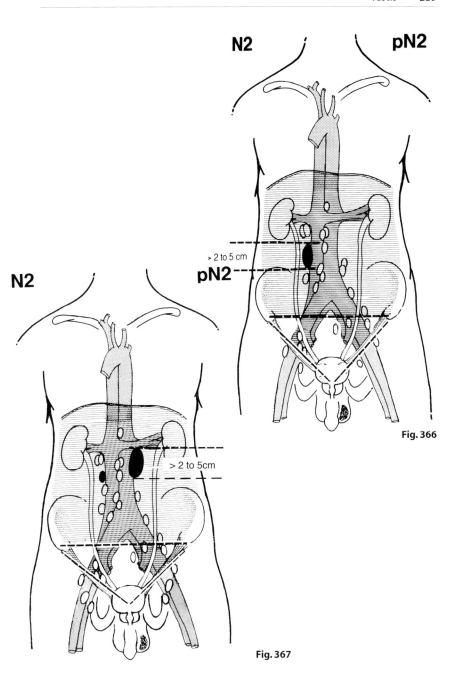

N2

pN2

> 2 to 5 cm

pN2

**Fig. 366**

N2

> 2 to 5 cm

**Fig. 367**

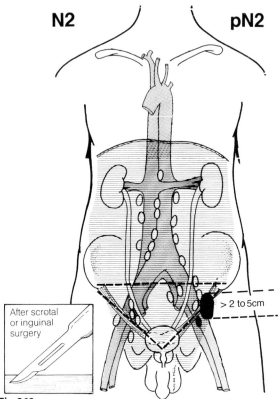

**N2**    **pN2**

After scrotal
or inguinal
surgery

> 2 to 5 cm

**Fig. 368**

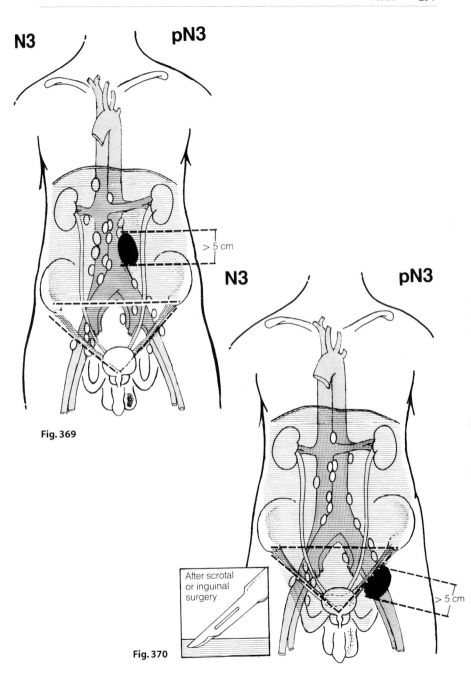

N3          pN3

> 5 cm

**Fig. 369**

N3          pN3

> 5 cm

After scrotal
or inguinal
surgery

**Fig. 370**

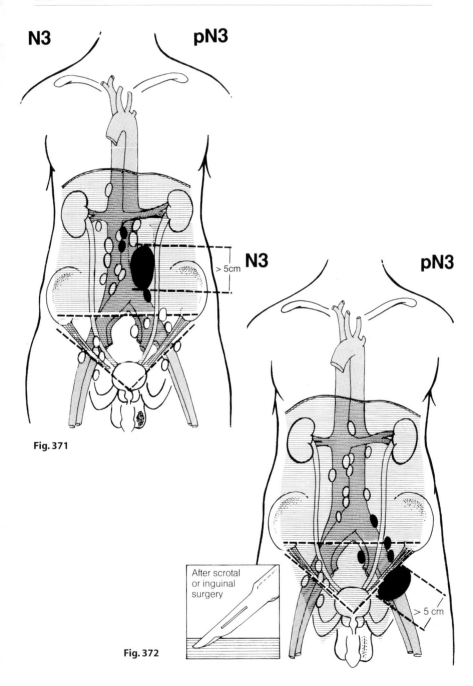

N3            pN3

N3            pN3

> 5cm

Fig. 371

After scrotal
or inguinal
surgery

Fig. 372

> 5 cm

# pTN Pathological Classification

## pT – Primary Tumour

pTX  Primary tumour cannot be assessed (if no radical orchiectomy has been performed TX is used)
pT0  No evidence of primary tumour, e.g. histological scar in testis
pTis  Intratubular germ cell neoplasia (carcinoma in situ)

pT1  Tumour limited to testis and epididymis without vascular/lymphatic invasion; tumour may invade tunica albuginea but not tunica vaginalis (Fig. 373)
pT2  Tumour limited to testis and epididymis with vascular/lymphatic invasion (Fig. 373) or tumour extending through tunica albuginea with involvement of tunica vaginalis (Fig. 374)

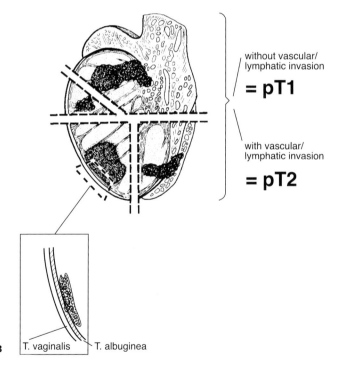

without vascular/
lymphatic invasion

= pT1

with vascular/
lymphatic invasion

= pT2

**Fig. 373**  T. vaginalis      T. albuginea

## pT2

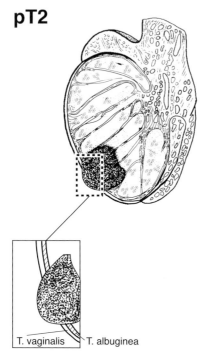

T. vaginalis    T. albuginea

**Fig. 374**

pT3   Tumour invades spermatic cord with or without vascular/lymphatic invasion (Fig. 375)

pT4   Tumour invades scrotum with or without vascular/lymphatic invasion (Fig. 376)

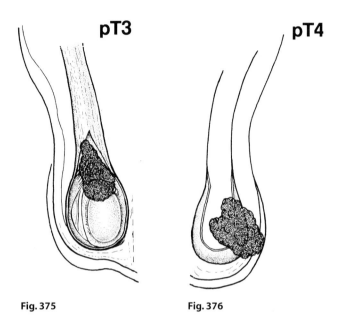

**pT3**   **pT4**

**Fig. 375**          **Fig. 376**

## pN – Regional Lymph Nodes

pNX   Regional lymph nodes cannot be assessed

pN0   No regional lymph node metastasis

pN1   Metastasis with a lymph node mass 2 cm or less in greatest dimension and 5 or fewer positive nodes, none more than 2 cm in greatest dimension (Figs. 360–363, pp. 284–286)

pN2   Metastasis with a lymph node mass more than 2 cm but not more than 5 cm in greatest dimension (Figs. 366–368, pp. 289–290); or more than 5 nodes positive, none more than 5 cm (Fig. 364, p. 287); or evidence of extranodal extension of tumour (Fig. 365, p. 288)

pN3   Metastasis with a lymph node mass more than 5 cm in greatest dimension (Figs. 369–372, p. 291–292)

# Kidney (ICD-O C64) (Fig. 377)

## Rules for Classification

The classification applies only to renal cell carcinoma. There should be histological confirmation of the disease.

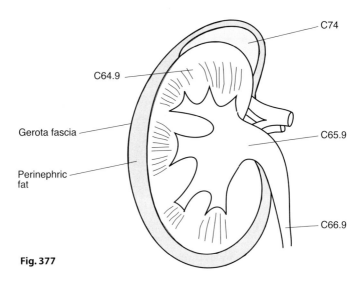

**Fig. 377**

## Regional Lymph Nodes (Fig. 378)

The regional lymph nodes are the hilar, abdominal para-aortic and paracaval nodes. Laterality does not affect the N categories.

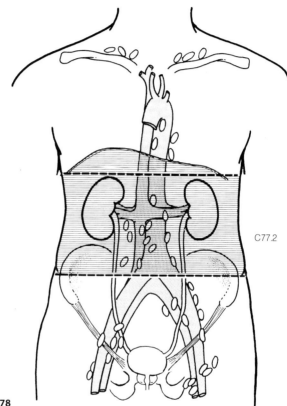

C77.2

**Fig. 378**

# TN Clinical Classification

## T – Primary Tumour

TX    Primary tumour cannot be assessed
T0    No evidence of primary tumour

T1    Tumour 7 cm or less in greatest dimension, limited to the kidney
      (Fig. 379)

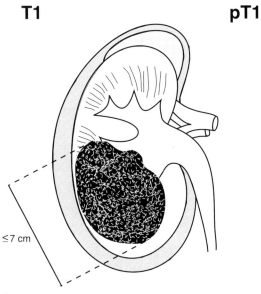

**T1**                              **pT1**

≤7 cm

**Fig. 379**

T2    Tumour more than 7 cm in greatest dimension, limited to the kidney (Fig. 380)

T3    Tumour extends into major veins or invades adrenal gland or perinephric tissues but not beyond Gerota fascia

    T3a    Tumour invades adrenal gland or perinephric tissues but not beyond Gerota fascia (Fig. 381)

    T3b    Tumour grossly extends into renal vein(s) or vena cava below diaphragm (Fig. 382)

    T3c    Tumour grossly extends into vena cava above diaphragm (Fig. 383)

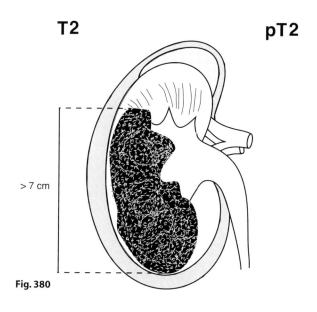

**T2**                    **pT2**

> 7 cm

**Fig. 380**

**T3a**

**T3a**

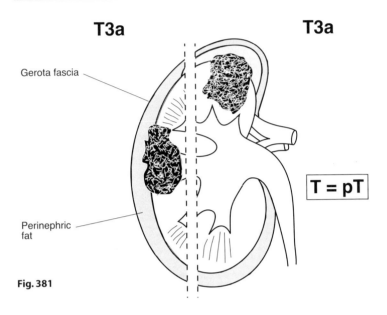

Gerota fascia

Perinephric fat

$T = pT$

**Fig. 381**

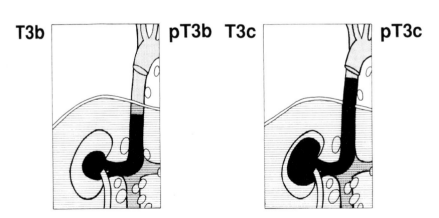

**T3b**          **pT3b**   **T3c**          **pT3c**

**Fig. 382**          **Fig. 383**

T4    Tumour invades beyond Gerota fascia (Fig. 384)

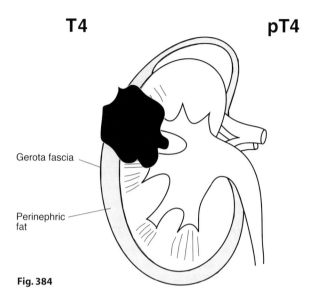

**T4**                                                            **pT4**

Gerota fascia

Perinephric
fat

**Fig. 384**

## N – Regional Lymph Nodes

NX    Regional lymph nodes cannot be assessed
N0    No regional lymph node metastasis
N1    Metastasis in a single regional lymph node (Fig. 385)
N2    Metastasis in more than one regional lymph node (Figs. 385, 386)

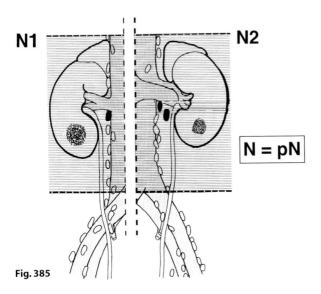

**N1**    **N2**

N = pN

**Fig. 385**

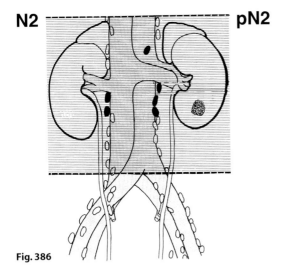

**N2**    **pN2**

**Fig. 386**

## pTN Pathological Classification

The pT and pN categories correspond to the T and N categories.

# Renal Pelvis and Ureter (ICD-O C65, C66)

## Rules for Classification

The classification applies only to carcinomas. Papilloma is excluded. There should be histological or cytological confirmation of the disease.

## Anatomical Sites (See Fig. 377, p. 296)

1. Renal pelvis (C65.9)
2. Ureter (C66.9)

## Regional Lymph Nodes (See Fig. 479, p. 371)

The regional lymph nodes are the hilar, abdominal para-aortic and paracaval nodes and, for ureter, intrapelvic nodes. Laterality does not affect the N classification.

## TN Clinical Classification

### T – Primary Tumour

TX    Primary tumour cannot be assessed
T0    No evidence of primary tumour
Ta    Non-invasive papillary carcinoma (Fig. 387)
Tis   Carcinoma in situ

T1    Tumour invades subepithelial connective tissue (Fig. 387)
T2    Tumour invades muscularis (Fig. 387)
T3    *(Renal pelvis)* Tumour invades beyond muscularis into peripelvic fat or renal parenchyma (Fig. 388)
      *(Ureter)* Tumour invades beyond muscularis into periureteric fat (Fig. 388)

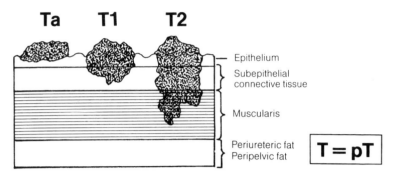

**Fig. 387**

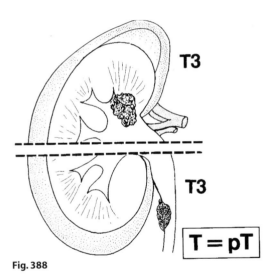

**Fig. 388**

T4    Tumour invades adjacent organs (Figs. 389, 390) or through the kidney into the perinephric fat (Fig. 391)

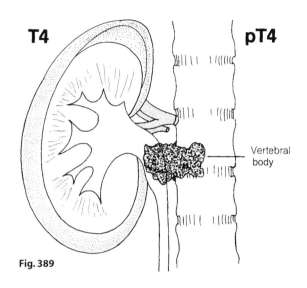

Fig. 389

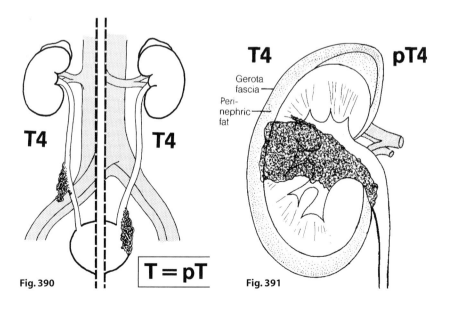

Fig. 390

Fig. 391

## N – Regional Lymph Nodes

NX    Regional lymph nodes cannot be assessed
N0    No regional lymph node metastasis
N1    Metastasis in a single lymph node, 2 cm or less in greatest dimension (Fig. 392)
N2    Metastasis in a single lymph node, more than 2 cm but not more than 5 cm in greatest dimension (Fig. 393), or multiple lymph nodes, none more than 5 cm in greatest dimension (Fig. 394)
N3    Metastasis in a lymph node, more than 5 cm in greatest dimension (Figs. 395, 396)

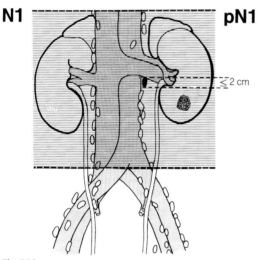

**N1**    **pN1**

$\leq 2$ cm

**Fig. 392**

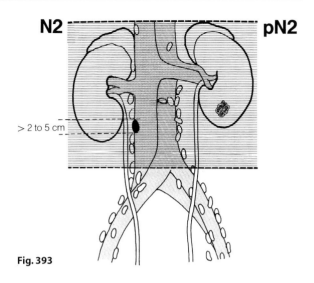

**Fig. 393**

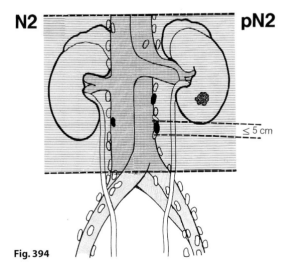

**Fig. 394**

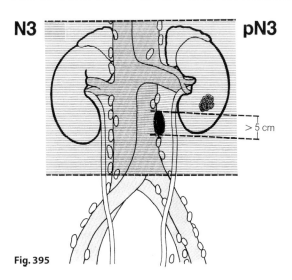

**Fig. 395**

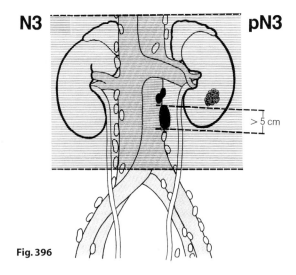

**Fig. 396**

## pTN Pathological Classification

The pT and pN categories correspond to the T and N categories.

# Urinary Bladder (ICD-O C67)

## Rules for Classification

The classification applies only to carcinomas. Papilloma is excluded. There should be histological or cytological confirmation of the disease.

## Anatomical Subsites (Fig. 397)

1. Trigone (C67.0)
2. Dome (C67.1)
3. Lateral wall (C67.2)
4. Anterior wall (C67.3)
5. Posterior wall (C67.4)
6. Bladder neck (C67.5)
7. Ureteric orifice (C67.6)
8. Urachus (C67.7)

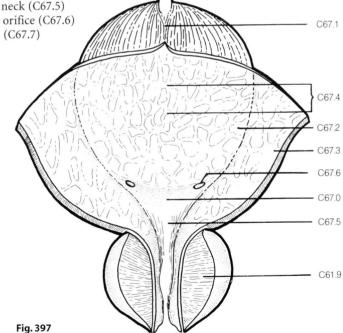

**Fig. 397**

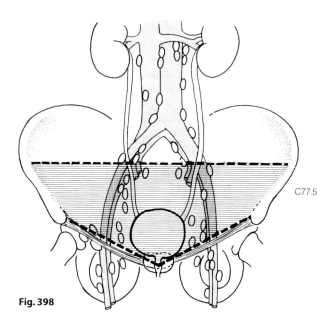

C77.5

**Fig. 398**

## Regional Lymph Nodes (Fig. 398)

The regional lymph nodes are the nodes of the true pelvis which essentially are the pelvic nodes below the bifurcation of the common iliac arteries. Laterality does not affect the N classification.

## TN Clinical Classification

### T – Primary Tumour (Fig. 399)

The suffix (m) should be added to the appropriate T category to indicate multiple tumours. The suffix (is) may be added to any T to indicate presence of associated carcinoma in situ.

| | |
|---|---|
| TX | Primary tumour cannot be assessed |
| T0 | No evidence of primary tumour |
| Ta | Non-invasive papillary carcinoma |
| Tis | Carcinoma in situ: "flat tumour" |

| T1 | Tumour invades subepithelial connective tissue |
| T2 | Tumour invades muscle |
| | T2a | Tumour invades superficial muscle (inner half) |
| | T2b | Tumour invades deep muscle (outer half) |
| T3 | Tumour invades perivesical tissue |
| | T3a | microscopically |
| | T3b | macroscopically (extravesical mass) |
| T4 | Tumour invades any of the following: prostate, uterus, vagina, pelvic wall, abdominal wall |
| | T4a | Tumour invades prostate or uterus or vagina |
| | T4b | Tumour invades pelvic wall or abdominal wall |

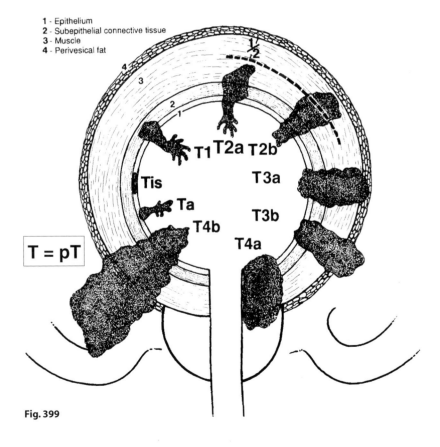

1 - Epithelium
2 - Subepithelial connective tissue
3 - Muscle
4 - Perivesical fat

**Fig. 399**

## N – Regional Lymph Nodes

NX    Regional lymph nodes cannot be assessed

N0    No regional lymph node metastasis

N1    Metastasis in a single lymph node, 2 cm or less in greatest dimension (Fig. 400)

N2    Metastasis in a single lymph node, more than 2 cm but not more than 5 cm in greatest dimension (Fig. 401); or multiple lymph nodes, none more than 5 cm in greatest dimension (Fig. 402)

N3    Metastasis in a lymph node, more than 5 cm in greatest dimension (Figs. 403, 404)

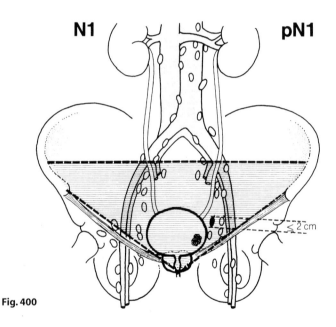

**Fig. 400**

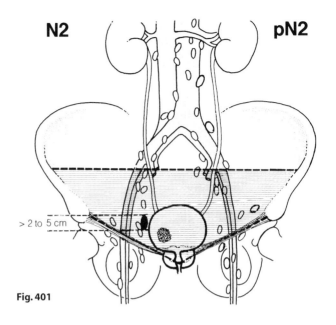

**N2**                    **pN2**

> 2 to 5 cm

**Fig. 401**

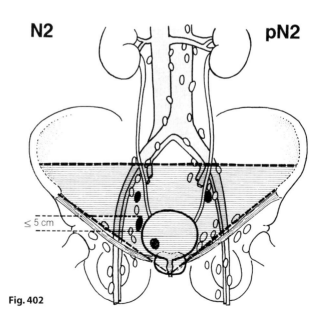

**N2**                    **pN2**

≤ 5 cm

**Fig. 402**

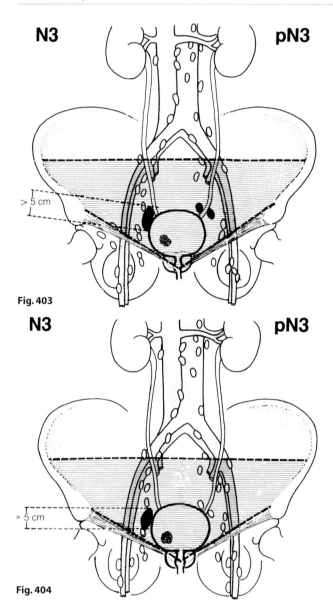

**N3**    **pN3**

**Fig. 403**

**N3**    **pN3**

**Fig. 404**

## pTN Pathological Classification

The pT and pN categories correspond to the T and N categories.

# Urethra

## Rules for Classification

The classification applies to carcinomas of the urethra (ICD-O C68.0) and transitional cell carcinomas of the prostate (ICD-O C61) and prostatic urethra. There should be histological or cytological confirmation of the disease.

## Regional Lymph Nodes (See Fig. 479, p. 371)

The regional lymph nodes are the inguinal and the pelvic lymph nodes. Laterality does not affect the N classification.

## TN Clinical Classification

### T – Primary Tumour

TX    Primary tumour cannot be assessed
T0    No evidence of primary tumour

*Urethra (male and female)*

Ta    Non-invasive papillary, polypoid or verrucous carcinoma (Figs. 405, 406)
Tis   Carcinoma in situ

T1    Tumour invades subepithelial connective tissue (Figs. 405, 407)
T2    Tumour invades any of the following: corpus spongiosum, prostate, periurethral muscle (Figs. 405, 408, 409)
T3    Tumour invades any of the following: corpus cavernosum, beyond prostatic capsule, anterior vagina, bladder neck (Figs. 410–412)
T4    Tumour invades other adjacent organs (Fig. 413)

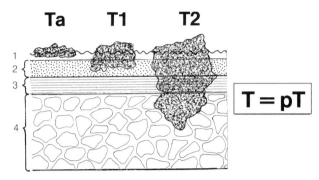

**Fig. 405.**   *1* Epithelium; *2* subepithelial connective tissue; *3* urethral muscle; *4* urogenital diaphragm

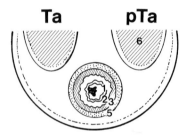

**Fig. 406.**   *1* Epithelium; *2* subepithelial connective tissue; *3* urethral muscle; *5* corpus spongiusm; *6* corpus cavernosum

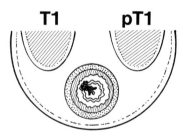

**Fig. 407**

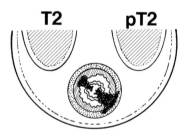

**Fig. 408**

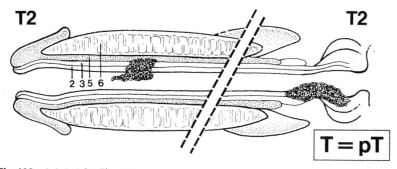

**Fig. 409.**  *2, 3, 5, 6:* See Fig. 406

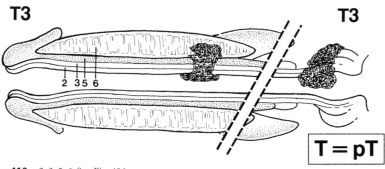

**Fig. 410.**  *2, 3, 5, 6:* See Fig. 406

**T3**                              **pT3**

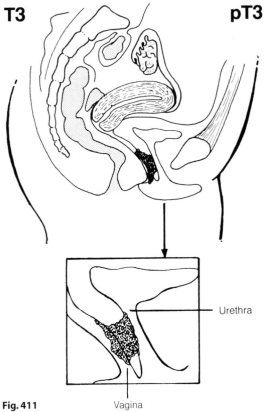

Urethra

**Fig. 411**          Vagina

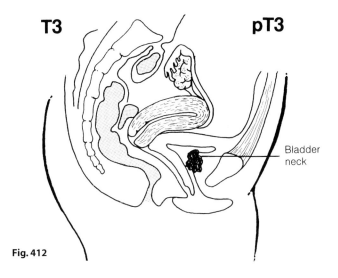

**T3**　　　　　　　　　**pT3**

Bladder
neck

**Fig. 412**

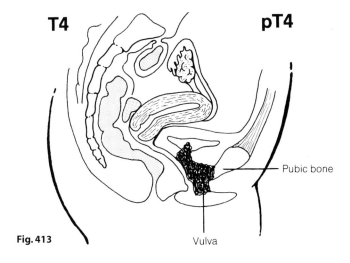

**T4**　　　　　　　　　**pT4**

Pubic bone

**Fig. 413**

Vulva

*Transitional cell carcinoma of prostate (prostatic urethra)*

Tis pu  Carcinoma in situ, involvement of prostatic urethra (Fig. 414)
Tis pd  Carcinoma in situ, involvement of prostatic ducts (Fig. 415)

T1      Tumour invades subepithelial connective tissue (Figs. 414, 415)
T2      Tumour invades any of the following: prostatic stroma, corpus spongio-
        sum, periurethral muscle (Figs. 415, 416)
T3      Tumour invades any of the following: corpus cavernosum, beyond
        prostatic capsule, bladder neck (extraprostatic extension) (Fig. 417)
T4      Tumour invades other adjacent organs (invasion of the bladder)
        (Fig. 418)

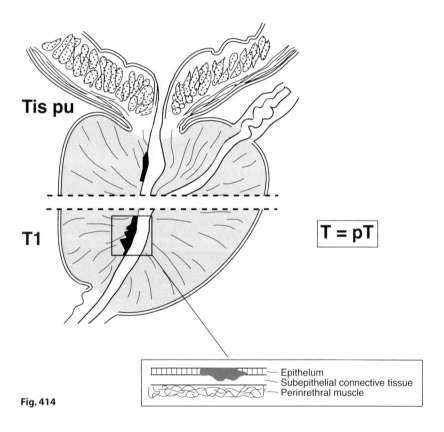

**Fig. 414**

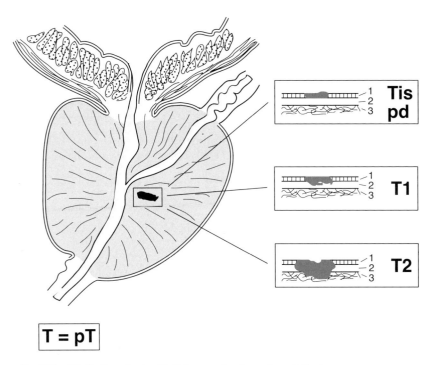

**Fig. 415.** *1* Epithelium, *2* subepithelial connective tissue, *3* prostatic stroma

**T2**　　　　　　　　　　　　**pT2**

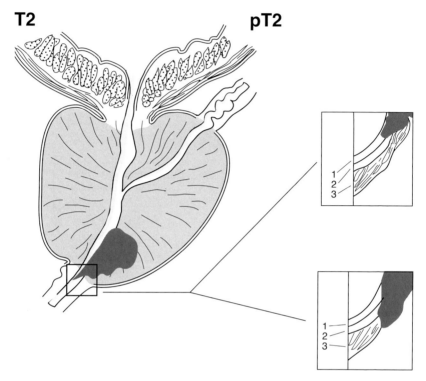

**Fig. 416.** *1* Urethral epithelium and subepithelial connective tissue, *2* periurethral muscle, *3* corpus spongiosum

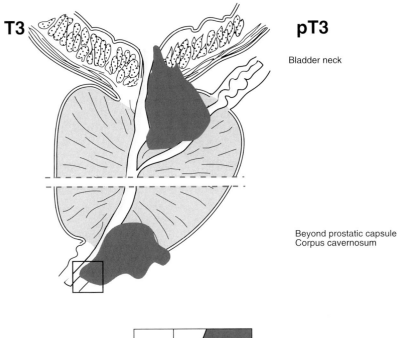

**T3**

**pT3**

Bladder neck

Beyond prostatic capsule
Corpus cavernosum

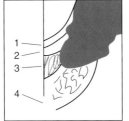

1 = Urethrol epithelum
     and connective tissue
2 = Perinrethral muscle
3 = Corpus spongiosum
4 =  orpus cavernosum

**Fig. 417**

# T4

# pT4

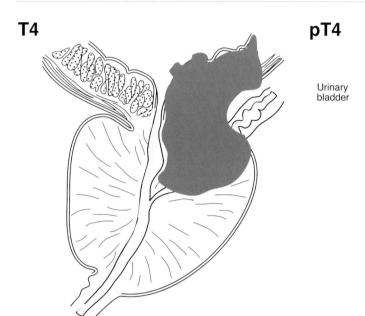

Urinary
bladder

**Fig. 418**

## N – Regional Lymph Nodes

NX   Regional lymph nodes cannot be assessed
N0   No regional lymph node metastasis
N1   Metastasis in a single lymph node, 2 cm or less in greatest dimension
     (Fig. 419)

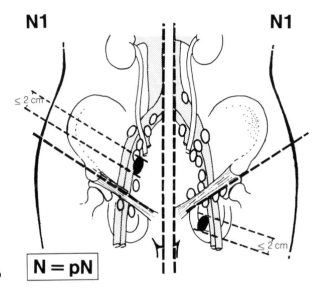

**Fig. 419**

N2     Metastasis in a single lymph node more than 2 cm in greatest dimension
       (Fig. 420), or multiple lymph nodes (Fig. 421)

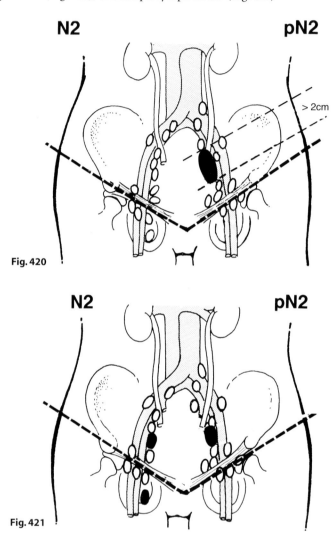

**Fig. 420**

**Fig. 421**

## pTN Pathological Classification

The pT and pN categories correspond to the T and N categories.

# Ophthalmic Tumours

## Introductory Notes

Tumours of the eye and its adnexa are a disparate group including carcinomas, melanoma, sarcomas and retinoblastoma. For clinical convenience they are presented in one section.

Tumours in the following sites are classified:

Eyelid (eyelid melanoma is classified with skin tumours)
Conjunctiva
Uvea
Retina
Orbit
Lacrimal gland

For histological nomenclature and diagnostic criteria, reference to the WHO classification [Zimmerman LE (1980) Histological typing of tumours of the eye and its adnexa. WHO, Geneva] is recommended.

## Regional Lymph Nodes (Fig. 422)

The regional lymph nodes are the preauricular *(1)*, submandibular *(2)* and cervical *(3)* lymph nodes.

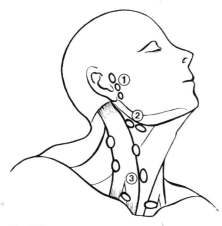

**Fig. 422**

The definitions of the N categories for ophthalmic tumours are:

### N – Regional Lymph Nodes

NX     Regional lymph nodes cannot be assessed
N0     No regional lymph node metastasis
N1     Regional lymph node metastasis

# Carcinoma of Eyelid (ICD-O C44.1)

## Rules for Classification

There should be histological confirmation of the disease and division of cases by histological type, e.g. basal cell, squamous cell, sebaceous carcinoma.

## T Clinical Classification

### T – Primary Tumour

TX    Primary tumour cannot be assessed
T0    No evidence of primary tumour
Tis   Carcinoma in situ

T1    Tumour of any size, not invading the tarsal plate; or at eyelid margin, 5 mm or less in greatest dimension (Fig. 423)

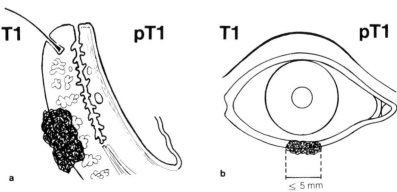

**Fig. 423a, b**

T2    Tumour invades tarsal plate; or at eyelid margin, more than 5 mm but not more than 10 mm in greatest dimension (Fig. 424)

T3    Tumour involves full eyelid thickness; or at eyelid margin, more than 10 mm in greatest dimension (Fig. 425)

T4    Tumour invades adjacent structures (Fig. 426)

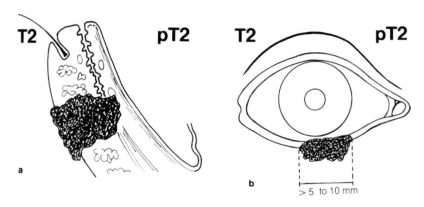

**Fig. 424a, b**

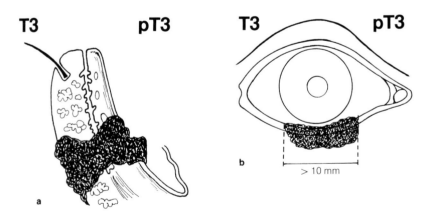

**Fig. 425a, b**

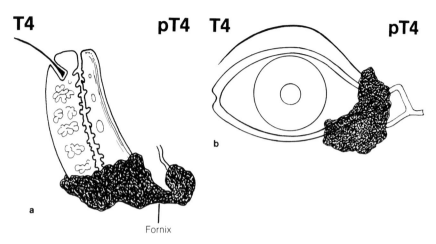

Fig. 426a, b

## pT Pathological Classification

The pT categories correspond to the T categories.

# Carcinoma of Conjunctiva (ICD-O C69.0)

## Rules for Classification

There should be histological confirmation of the disease and division of cases by histological type, e.g. mucoepidermoid and squamous cell carcinoma.

## T Clinical Classification

### T – Primary Tumour

TX    Primary tumour cannot be assessed
T0    No evidence of primary tumour
Tis   Carcinoma in situ

T1    Tumour 5 mm or less in greatest dimension (Fig. 427)
T2    Tumour more than 5 mm in greatest dimension, without invasion of adjacent structures (Fig. 428)
T3    Tumour invades adjacent structures, excluding the orbit (Fig. 429)
T4    Tumour invades the orbit (Fig. 430)

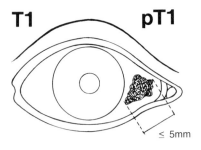

**Fig. 427**

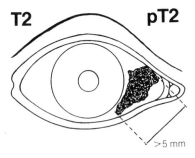

**Fig. 428**

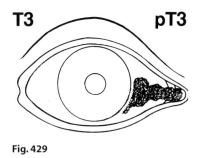

Fig. 429

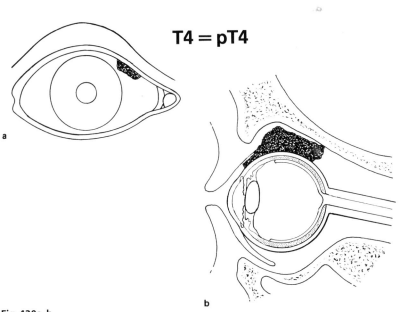

Fig. 430a, b

## pT Pathological Classification

The pT categories correspond to the T categories.

# Malignant Melanoma of Conjunctiva (ICD-O C69.0)

## Rules for Classification

The classification applies only to malignant melanoma. There should be histological confirmation of the disease. The tumour should be distinguished from non-tumorous pigmentation.

## T Clinical Classification

### T – Primary Tumour

TX     Primary tumour cannot be assessed
T0     No evidence of primary tumour

T1     Tumour(s) of bulbar conjunctiva occupying one quadrant or less (Fig 431)

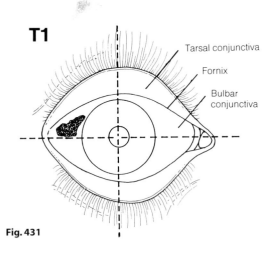

**T1**

Tarsal conjunctiva

Fornix

Bulbar conjunctiva

**Fig. 431**

T2    Tumour(s) of bulbar conjunctiva occupying more than one quadrant (Fig. 432)

T3    Tumour(s) of conjunctival fornix and/or palpebral conjunctiva and/or caruncle (Fig. 433)

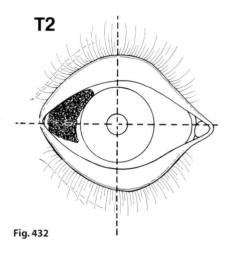

**Fig. 432**

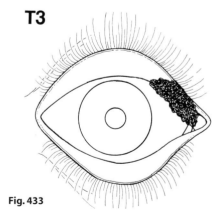

**Fig. 433**

T4    Tumour invades eyelid, cornea and/or orbit (Fig. 434)

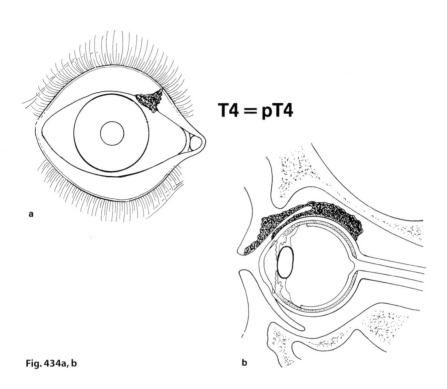

**T4 = pT4**

**Fig. 434a, b**

a

b

## pT Pathological Classification

### pT – Primary Tumour

pTX    Primary tumour cannot be assessed
pT0    No evidence of primary tumour

pT1    Tumour(s) of the bulbar conjunctiva occupying one quadrant or less and 2 mm or less in thickness (Fig. 435)
pT2    Tumour(s) of the bulbar conjunctiva occupying more than one quadrant and 2 mm or less in thickness (Fig. 435)

pT3    Tumour(s) of the conjunctival fornix and/or palpebral conjunctiva and/ or caruncle or tumour of the bulbar conjunctiva more than 2 mm in thickness (Fig. 436)

pT4    Tumour invades eyelid, cornea and/or orbit (Fig. 434)

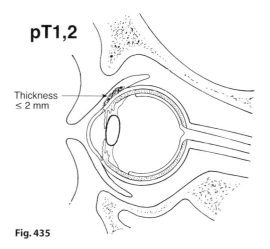

**Fig. 435**

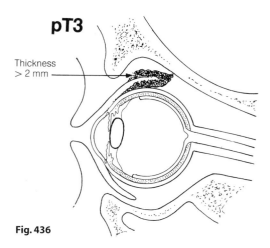

**Fig. 436**

# Malignant Melanoma of Uvea (ICD-O C69.3,4)

## Rules for Classification

There should be histological confirmation of the disease.

## Anatomical Sites

1. Iris (C69.4)
2. Ciliary body (C69.4)
3. Choroid (C69.3)

## T Clinical Classification

### T – Primary Tumour

TX    Primary tumour cannot be assessed
T0    No evidence of primary tumour

### *Iris*

T1    Tumour limited to the iris (Fig. 437)
T2    Tumour involves one quadrant or less, with invasion into anterior cham-
      ber angle (Fig. 438)

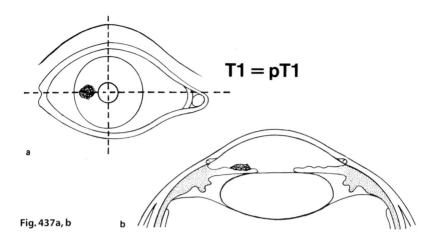

**T1 = pT1**

**Fig. 437a, b**

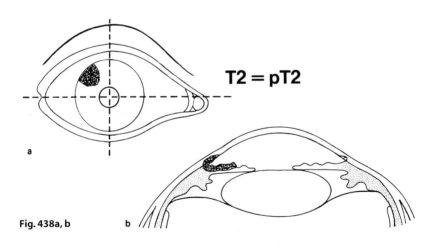

**T2 = pT2**

**Fig. 438a, b**

T3    Tumour involves more than one quadrant, with invasion into anterior chamber angle, ciliary body, and/or choroid (Figs. 439, 440)

T4    Tumour with extraocular extension (Fig. 441)

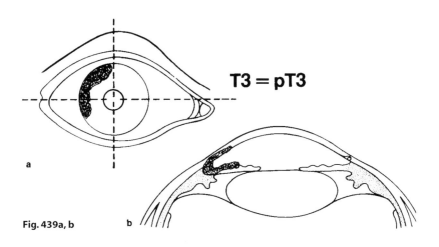

**T3 = pT3**

**Fig. 439a, b**

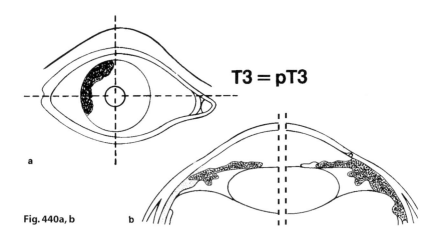

**T3 = pT3**

**Fig. 440a, b**

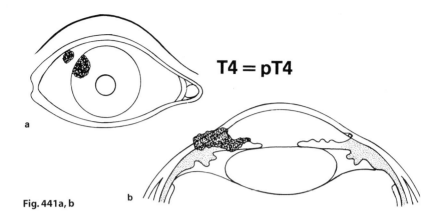

T4 = pT4

a

b

**Fig. 441a, b**

*Ciliary Body*

T1     Tumour limited to the ciliary body (Fig. 442)
T2     Tumour invades anterior chamber and/or iris (Fig. 443)
T3     Tumour invades choroid (Fig. 444)
T4     Tumour with extraocular extension (Fig. 445)

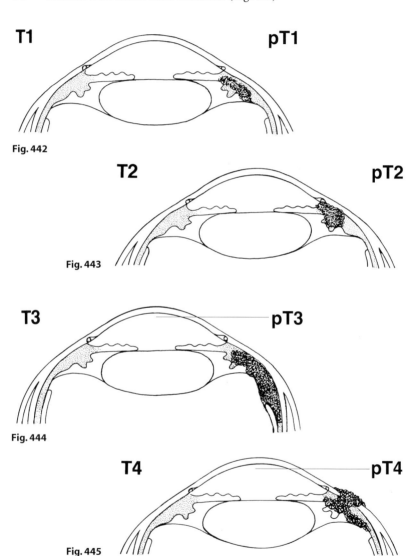

**T1**                                          **pT1**

**Fig. 442**

**T2**                                          **pT2**

**Fig. 443**

**T3**                                          **pT3**

**Fig. 444**

**T4**                                          **pT4**

**Fig. 445**

*Choroid*

T1    Tumour 10 mm or less in greatest dimension with an elevation 3 mm or less[1]

    T1a    Tumour 7 mm or less in greatest dimension with an elevation 2 mm or less (Fig. 446)

    T1b    Tumour more than 7 mm but not more than 10 mm in greatest dimension with an elevation more than 2 mm but not more than 3 mm (Fig. 447)

T2    Tumour more than 10 mm but not more than 15 mm in greatest dimension with an elevation more than 3 mm but not more than 5 mm (Fig. 448)

**Note:**    1. When dimension and elevation show a difference in classification, the highest category should be used for classification. The tumour base may be estimated in optic disc diameters (dd, average 1 dd = 1.5 mm) and the elevation in dioptres (average 3 dioptres = 1 mm); other techniques, such as ultrasonography and computerized stereometry, may provide a more accurate measurement.

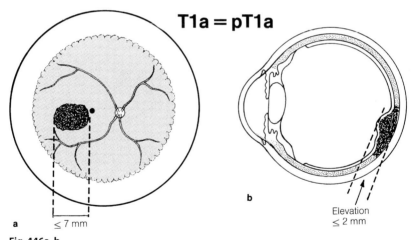

**T1a = pT1a**

a    ≤ 7 mm

b    Elevation ≤ 2 mm

**Fig. 446a, b**

# T1b = pT1b

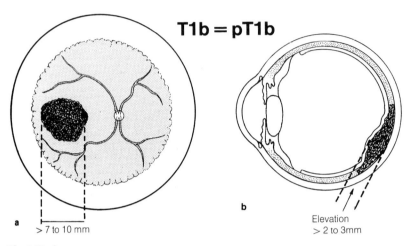

**a**  |— > 7 to 10 mm

**b**

Elevation
> 2 to 3mm

**Fig. 447a, b**

# T2 = pT2

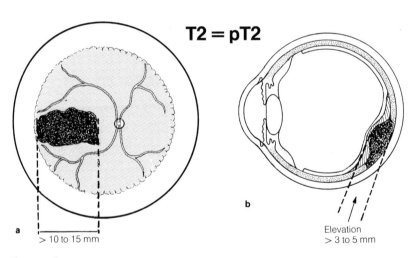

**a**  |— > 10 to 15 mm

**b**

Elevation
> 3 to 5 mm

**Fig. 448a, b**

T3    Tumour more than 15 mm in greatest dimension or with an elevation
      more than 5 mm (Fig. 449)
T4    Tumour with extraocular extension (Fig. 450)

**Note:**    See p. 341.

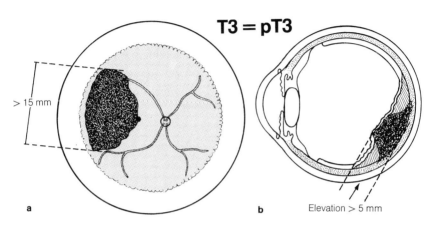

**Fig. 449a, b**

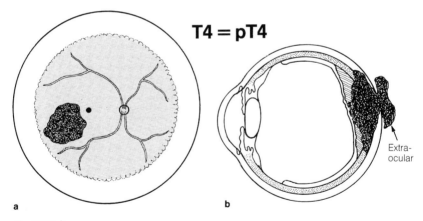

**Fig. 450a, b**

## pT Pathological Classification

The pT categories correspond to the T categories.

# Retinoblastoma (ICD-O C69.2)

## Rules for Classification

In bilateral cases, each eye should be classified separately. The classification does not apply to complete spontaneous regression of the tumour. There should be histological confirmation of the disease in an enucleated eye.

## T Clinical Classification

### T – Primary Tumour

The extent of retinal involvement is indicated as a percentage.

TX     Primary tumour cannot be assessed
T0     No evidence of primary tumour

T1     Tumour(s) limited to 25% of the retina or less (Fig. 451)

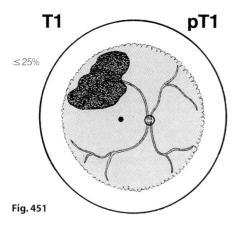

**Fig. 451**

T2    Tumour(s) involve(s) more than 25% but not more than 50% of the retina (Fig. 452)

T3    Tumour(s) involve(s) more than 50% of the retina and/or invade(s) beyond the retina but remain(s) intraocular

    T3a    Tumour(s) involve(s) more than 50% of the retina and/or tumour cells in the vitreous body (Fig. 453)

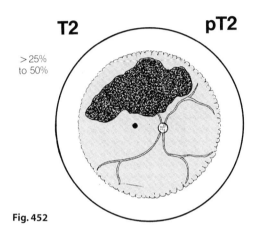

**T2**                            **pT2**

> 25% to 50%

**Fig. 452**

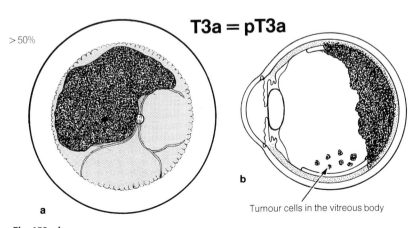

**T3a = pT3a**

> 50%

Tumour cells in the vitreous body

**a**         **b**

**Fig. 453a, b**

T3b    Tumour(s) involve(s) optic disc (Fig. 454)
T3c    Tumour(s) involve(s) anterior chamber and/or uvea (Fig. 455)

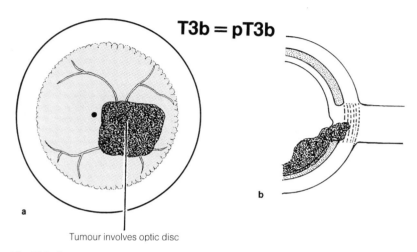

**Fig. 454a, b**

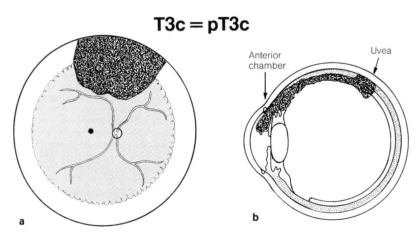

**Fig. 455a, b**

T4    Tumour with extraocular invasion (Figs. 456, 457)
    T4a    Tumour invades retrobulbar optic nerve (Fig. 456)
    T4b    Extraocular extension other than invasion of optic nerve
          (Fig. 457)

**Note:**  The following suffixes may be added to the appropriate T categories:
    (m) to indicate multiple tumours, e.g. T2(m)
    (f)  to indicate cases with a known family history
    (d) to indicate diffuse retinal involvement without the formation of
        discrete masses

**T4**

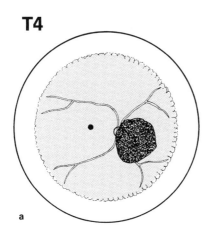

a

**T4a=pT4a**                **T4a=pT4b**

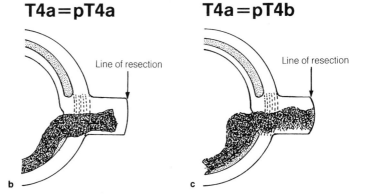

b                     c

**Fig. 456a–c**

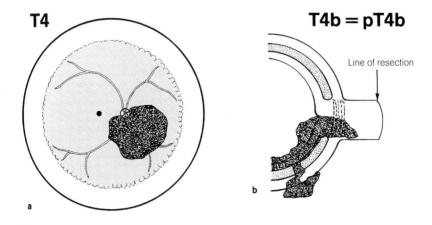

**Fig. 457a, b**

## pT Pathological Classification

### pT – Primary Tumour

pTX　Primary tumour cannot be assessed
pT0　No evidence of primary tumour

pT1　Corresponds to T1 (Fig. 451, see p. 346)
pT2　Corresponds to T2 (Fig. 452, see p. 347)
pT3　Corresponds to T3
　　　pT3a　Corresponds to T3a (Fig. 453, see p. 347)
　　　pT3b　Tumour invades optic nerve as far as lamina cribrosa
　　　　　　(Fig. 454, see p. 348)
　　　pT3c　Tumour in anterior chamber and/or invasion with thickening of
　　　　　　uvea and/or intrascleral invasion (Fig. 455, see p. 348)
pT4　Corresponds to T4
　　　pT4a　Intraneural tumour beyond lamina cribrosa, but not at line of
　　　　　　resection (Fig. 456, see p. 349)
　　　pT4b　Tumour at line of resection or other extraocular extension
　　　　　　(Figs. 456c, 457b)

# Sarcoma of Orbit (ICD-O C69.6)

## Rules for Classification

The classification applies only to sarcomas of soft tissue and bone. There should be histological confirmation of the disease and division of cases by histological type.

## T Clinical Classification

### T – Primary Tumour

TX    Primary tumour cannot be assessed
T0    No evidence of primary tumour

T1    Tumour 15 mm or less in greatest dimension (Fig. 458)
T2    Tumour more than 15 mm in greatest dimension (Fig. 459)
T3    Tumour of any size with diffuse invasion of orbital tissues and/or bony walls (Fig. 460)
T4    Tumour invades beyond the orbit to adjacent sinuses and/or to cranium (Fig. 461)

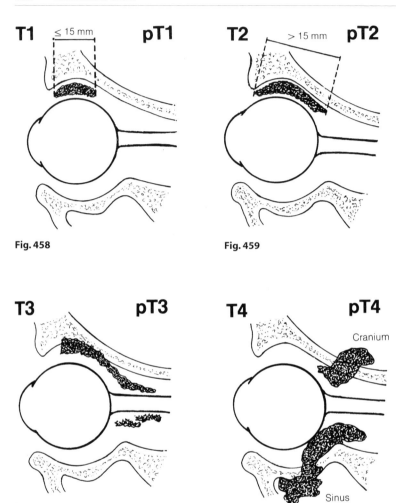

Fig. 458

Fig. 459

Fig. 460

Fig. 461

## pT Pathological Classification

The pT categories correspond to the T categories.

# Carcinoma of Lacrimal Gland (ICD-O C69.5)

## Rules for Classification

There should be histological confirmation of the disease and division of cases by histological type.

## T Clinical Classification

### T – Primary Tumour

TX   Primary tumour cannot be assessed
T0   No evidence of primary tumour

T1   Tumour 2.5 cm or less in greatest dimension, limited to the lacrimal gland (Fig. 462)
T2   Tumour 2.5 cm or less in greatest dimension, invading the periosteum of the fossa of the lacrimal gland (Fig. 463)

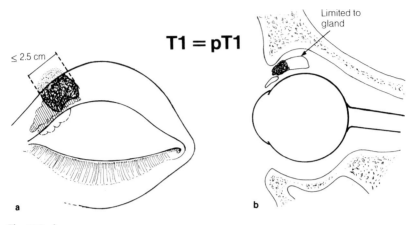

**T1 = pT1**

Limited to gland

≤ 2.5 cm

a    b

**Fig. 462a, b**

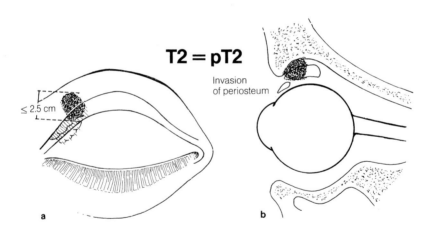

**T2 = pT2**

Invasion of periosteum

≤ 2.5 cm

a    b

**Fig. 463a, b**

T3   Tumour more than 2.5 cm but not more than 5 cm in greatest dimension (Fig. 464a)

    T3a   Tumour limited to the lacrimal gland (Fig. 464b)

    T3b   Tumour invades the periosteum of the fossa of the lacrimal gland (Fig. 464c)

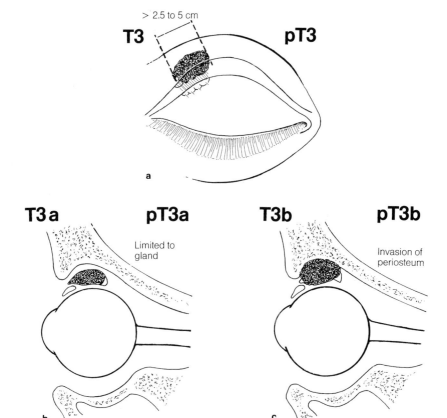

Fig. 464a–c

T4   Tumour more than 5 cm in greatest dimension (Fig. 465a)
   T4a   Tumour invades orbital soft tissues, optic nerve or globe, but *without* bone invasion (Fig. 465b)
   T4b   Tumour invades orbital soft tissues, optic nerve or globe, *with* bone invasion (Fig. 465c)

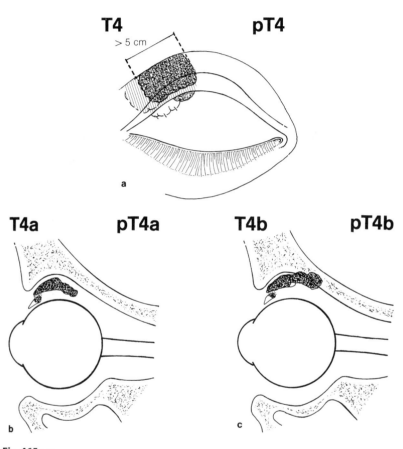

Fig. 465a–c

## pT Pathological Classification

The pT categories correspond to the T categories.

# Hodgkin Disease

## Introductory Notes

At the present time it is not considered practical to propose a TNM classification for Hodgkin disease.

Following the development of the Ann Arbor Classification for Hodgkin disease in 1971, the significance of two important observations with major impact on staging has been appreciated. First, extralymphatic disease, if localized and related to adjacent lymph node disease, does not adversely affect the survival of patients. Secondly, laparotomy with splenectomy has been introduced as a method for obtaining more information on the extent of the disease within the abdomen.

A stage classification based on information from histopathological examination of the spleen and lymph nodes obtained at laparotomy or laparoscopy cannot be compared with another without such exploration. Therefore, two systems of classification are presented, a clinical (cS) and a pathological (pS).

## Clinical Staging (cS)

Although recognized as incomplete, this is easily performed and should be reproducible from one centre to another. It is determined by history, clinical examination, imaging, blood analysis and the initial biopsy report. Bone marrow biopsy must be taken from a clinically or radiologically non-involved area of bone.

**Liver Involvement.** Clinical evidence of liver involvement must include either enlargement of the liver and at least an abnormal serum alkaline phosphatase level and two different liver function test abnormalities, or an abnormal liver demonstrated by imaging and one abnormal liver function test.

**Spleen Involvement.** Clinical evidence of spleen involvement is accepted if there is palpable enlargement of the spleen confirmed by imaging.

**Lymphatic and Extralymphatic Disease.** The lymphatic structures are as follows:

| | |
|---|---|
| Lymph nodes | Waldeyer ring |
| Spleen | Appendix |
| Thymus | Peyer patches |

The lymph nodes are grouped into regions, and one or more (2, 3 etc.) may be involved. The spleen is designated S and extralymphatic organs or sites E.

**Lung involvement** limited to one lobe, or perihilar extension associated with ipsilateral lymphadenopathy, or unilateral pleural effusion with or without lung involvement but with hilar lymphadenopathy are considered as localized extralymphatic diseases.

**Liver involvement** is always considered as *diffuse* extralymphatic disease

## Pathological Staging (pS)

This takes into account additional data and has a higher degree of precision. It should be applied whenever possible. A - (minus) or + (plus) sign should be added to the various symbols for the examined tissues, depending on the results of histopathological examination.

## Histopathological Information

This is classified by notations indicating the tissue sampled. The following notation is common to the distant metastases (or M1 categories) of all regions classified by the TNM system. However, in order to conform with the Ann Arbor classification, the initial letters used in that system are also given.

| | | | |
|---|---|---|---|
| Pulmonary | PUL or L | Bone marrow | MAR or M |
| Osseous | OSS or O | Pleura | PLE or P |
| Hepatic | HEP or H | Peritoneum | PER |
| Brain | BRA | Adrenals | ADR |
| Lymph nodes | LYM or N | Skin | SKI or D |
| | Other | OTH | |

## Clinical Stages (cS)

Stage I     Involvement of a single lymph node region (I) (Figs. 466-469), or loca-
            lized involvement of a single extralymphatic organ or site ($I_E$)
            (Fig. 470)

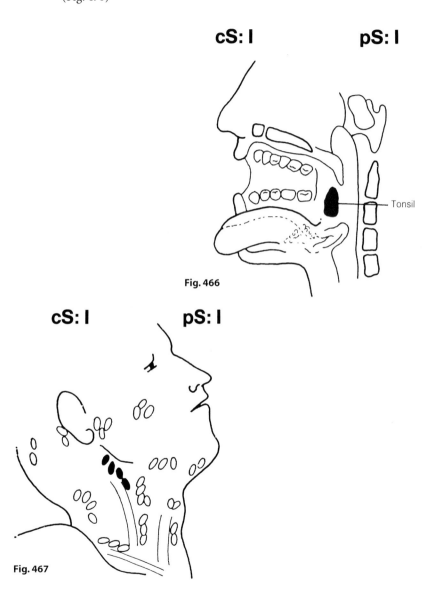

**cS: I**          **pS: I**

Tonsil

**Fig. 466**

**cS: I**          **pS: I**

**Fig. 467**

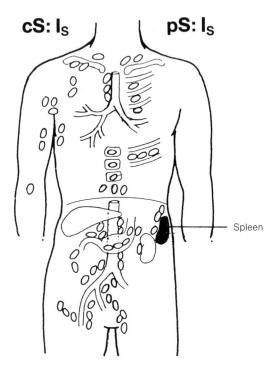

**cS: I_S**     **pS: I_S**

Spleen

**Fig. 468**

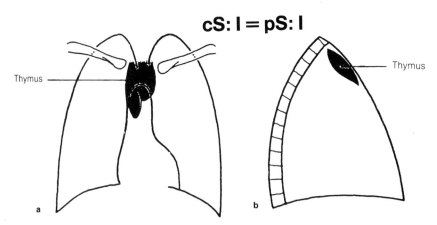

**cS: I = pS: I**

Thymus

Thymus

a

b

**Fig. 469a, b**

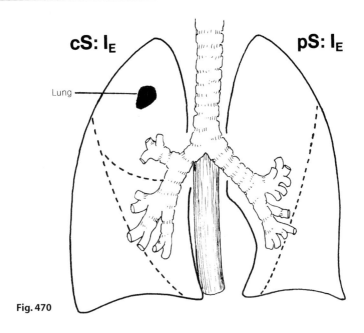

cS: I<sub>E</sub>

pS: I<sub>E</sub>

Lung

**Fig. 470**

Stage II   Involvement of two or more lymph node regions on the same side of the diaphragm (II) (Fig. 471), or localized involvement of a single extralymphatic organ or site and its regional lymph node(s) with or without involvement of other lymph node regions on the same side of the diaphragm ($II_E$) (Fig. 472)

**Note:**   The number of lymph node regions involved may be indicated by a subscript (e.g. $II_5$).

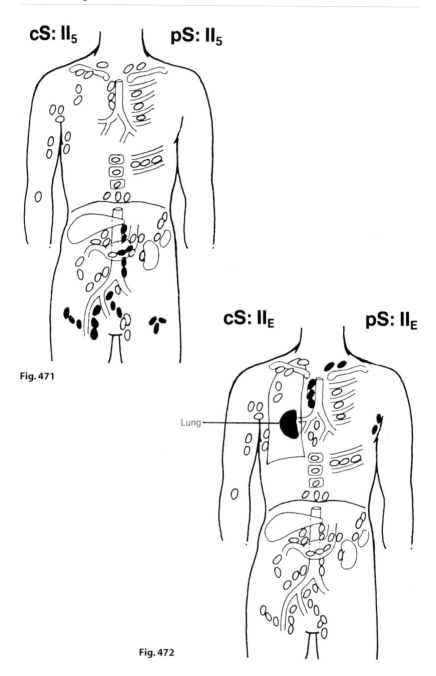

cS: II₅    pS: II₅

**Fig. 471**

cS: IIₑ    pS: IIₑ

Lung

**Fig. 472**

Stage III Involvement of lymph node regions on both sides of the diaphragm
(III) (Fig. 473), which may also be accompanied by localized involvement of an associated extralymphatic organ or site ($III_E$) (Fig. 474), or
by involvement of the spleen ($III_S$), or both $III_{E+S}$) (Fig. 475)

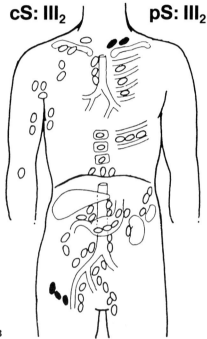

cS: $III_2$    pS: $III_2$

**Fig. 473**

**cS: III$_E$**

**pS: III$_E$**

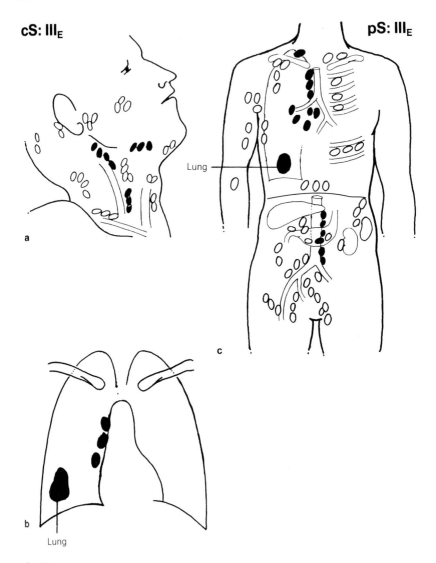

Lung

Lung

**Fig. 474a–c**

# cS: III$_{E+S}$ = pS: III$_{E+S}$

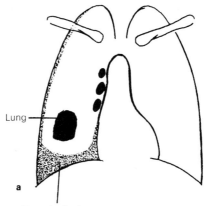

Lung

Pleural effusion

a

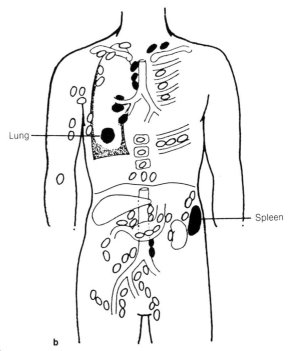

Lung

Spleen

b

**Fig. 475a, b**

Stage IV  Disseminated (multifocal) involvement of one or more extralymphatic organs, with or without associated lymph node involvement (Figs. 476, 477); or isolated extralymphatic organ involvement with distant (non-regional) nodal involvement (Fig. 478)

**Note:**    The site of Stage IV disease is identified further by specifying sites according to the notations listed on p. 358.

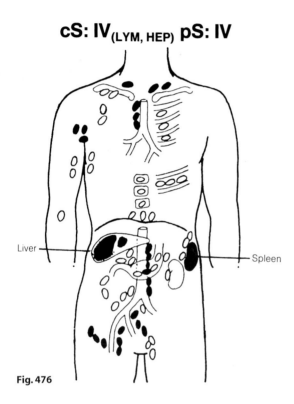

cS: IV(LYM, HEP) pS: IV

Liver

Spleen

**Fig. 476**

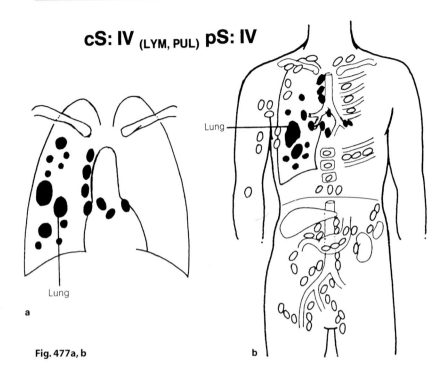

**Fig. 477a, b**

## A and B Classification (Symptoms)

Each stage should be divided into A and B according to the absence or presence of defined general symptoms. These are:

1. Unexplained weight loss of more than 10% of the usual body weight in the 6 months prior to first attendance
2. Unexplained fever with temperature above 38° C
3. Night sweats

**Note:** Pruritus alone does not qualify for B classification, nor does a short, febrile illness associated with a known infection.

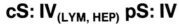

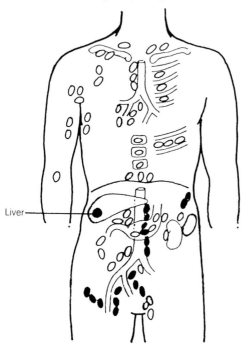

Liver

## Pathological Stages (pS)

The definitions of the four stages follow the same criteria as the clinical stages but with the additional information obtained following laparotomy or laparoscopy. Splenectomy, liver biopsy, lymph node biopsy and marrow biopsy are mandatory for the establishment of pathological stages. The results of these biopsies are recorded as indicated above (see p. 358 and Figs. 466–478, pp. 359–368).

# Non Hodgkin Lymphomas

As in Hodgkin disease, at the present time it is not considered practical to propose a TNM classification for non-Hodgkin lymphomas. Since no other convincing and tested staging system is available, the Ann Arbor classification is recommended with the same modification as for Hodgkin disease (see p. 357 and Figs. 466–478, pp. 359–368).

# Areas of Regional Lymph Nodes (Fig. 479)

| | |
|---|---|
| A↑[1] | Head and neck, cervical oesophagus, ophthalmic tumours |
| A-B[2] | Lung, pleural mesothelioma |
| A-B[3] | Intrathoracic oesophagus |
| B-C (partly) | Stomach |
| B-C (partly) | Liver, gallbladder, extrahepatic bile ducts, ampulla of Vater, pancreas, small intestine |
| B-C | Kidney, renal pelvis |
| B-C[4] | Colon |
| B-E | Ureter |
| B-C[5] | Testis |
| B-E and E↓ | Ovary, fallopian tube |
| C-E (partly)[6] | Rectum |
| C-E[7] | Corpus uteri, cervix uteri, upper two-thirds of vagina |
| D-E | Urinary bladder, prostate |
| D-E and E↓ | Penis, urethra |
| D-E (partly) and E↓ | Anal canal |
| E↓ | Lower third of vagina, vulva |
| F[8] | Breast |
| Skin | See Figs. 233–239 pp. 180–186. |

---

[1] Plus the upper anterior mediastinal lymph nodes for thyroid tumours.

[2] Plus the scalene and supraclavicular lymph nodes.

[3] Plus perigastric nodes (excluding coeliac nodes).

[4] Plus lymph nodes located inferior to the level of the aorta bifurcation, along the branching of the ileocolic and sigmoid arteries.

[5] Plus nodes along the spermatic vein. After previous scrotal or inguinal operations, the intrapelvic (C–E) and inguinal lymph nodes (E↓) are also considered as regional lymph nodes.

[6] The lymph nodes along the trunk of the inferior mesenteric artery are also considered as regional lymph nodes.

[7] For corpus uteri plus para-aortic nodes.

[8] Plus the ipsilateral internal mammary lymph nodes.

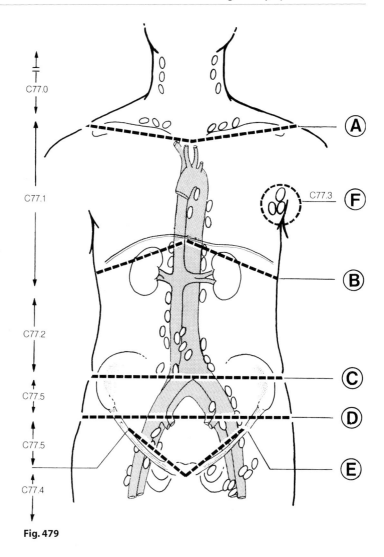

**Fig. 479**

Printing: Appl, Wemding
Binding: Appl, Wemding

# Springer
# and the
# environment

At Springer we firmly believe that an international science publisher has a special obligation to the environment, and our corporate policies consistently reflect this conviction.

We also expect our business partners – paper mills, printers, packaging manufacturers, etc. – to commit themselves to using materials and production processes that do not harm the environment. The paper in this book is made from low- or no-chlorine pulp and is acid free, in conformance with international standards for paper permanency.

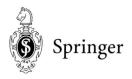 Springer